KU-515-535

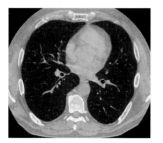

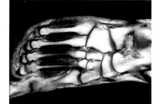

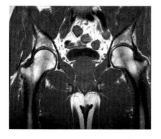

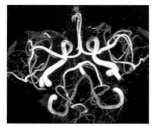

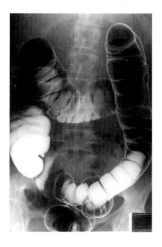

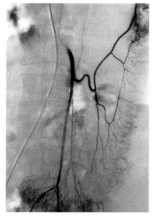

Imaging Atlas of
Human
Anatomy

Commissioning Editor: Richard Furn
Project Development Manager: Barbara Simmons
Project Manager: Colin Arthur
Designer: George Ajayi

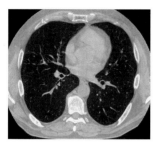
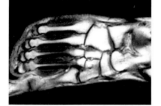
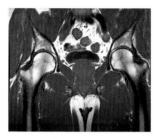
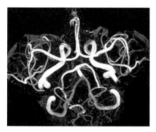

Imaging Atlas of Human Anatomy

Third Edition

Jamie Weir MBBS DMRD FRCP(Ed) FRANZCR (Hon) FRCR

Clinical Professor of Radiology, Grampian University Hospitals Trust, Aberdeen, UK

Peter H Abrahams MBBS FRCS(Ed) FRCR DO (Hon)

Professor of Clinical Anatomy, Kigezi International School of Medicine, Cambridge, UK, and St George's University, Grenada, West Indies

Fellow, Girton College, Cambridge, UK
Examiner to The Royal College of Surgeons of Edinburgh, Scotland
Family Practitioner, Brent, London, UK

With four contributors

Anna-Maria Belli MBBS DMRD FRCR

Consultant Radiologist and Senior Lecturer, St George's Hospital and Medical School, London, UK

Margaret D Hourihan MB BCh FRCR

Consultant Neuroradiologist, Department of Radiology, University Hospital of Wales, Cardiff, UK

Niall R Moore MA MB BChir FRCP FRCR

University Lecturer in Radiology, University of Oxford, UK
Honorary Consultant Radiologist, Oxford Radcliffe Hospital, UK

J Philip Owen MBBS DMRD FRCR

Senior Lecturer/Head of Department, University Department of Radiology, The University of Newcastle upon Tyne
Honorary Consultant in Radiology, Royal Victoria Infirmary, Newcastle upon Tyne, UK

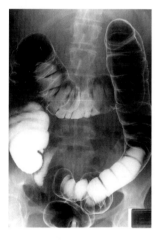
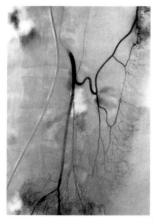

Mosby

Edinburgh   London   New York   Oxford
Philadelphia   St Louis   Sydney   Toronto 2003

MOSBY
An affiliate of Elsevier Science

© 2003, Elsevier Science Limited. All rights reserved.

The right of Jamie Weir and Peter H Abrahams to be identified as authors of this work has been asserted by them in accordance with the Copyright, Designs and Patents Act 1988.

No part of this publication may be reproduced, stored in a retrieval system, or transmitted in any form or by any means, electronic, mechanical, photocopying, recording or otherwise, without either the prior permission of the publishers or a licence permitting restricted copying in the United Kingdom issued by the Copyright Licensing Agency, 90 Tottenham Court Road, London W1T 4LP. Permissions may be sought directly from Elsevier's Health Sciences Rights Department in Philadelphia, USA: phone: (+1) 215 238 7869, fax: (+1) 215 238 2239, e-mail: healthpermissions@elsevier.com. You may also complete your request on-line via the Elsevier Science homepage (http://www.elsevier.com), by selecting 'Customer Support' and then 'Obtaining Permissions'.

First published 1997
Reprinted 2000
Reprinted 2001

Standard edition ISBN 0 7234 3221 2
International student edition ISBN 0 7234 3294 5

British Library Cataloguing in Publication Data
A catalogue record for this book is available from the British Library

Library of Congress Cataloging in Publication Data
A catalog record for this book is available from the Library of Congress

Notice
Medical knowledge is constantly changing. Standard safety precautions must be followed, but as new research and clinical experience broaden our knowledge, changes in treatment and drug therapy may become necessary or appropriate. Readers are advised to check the most current product information provided by the manufacturer of each drug to be administered to verify the recommended dose, the method and duration of administration, and contraindications. It is the responsibility of the practitioner, relying on experience and knowledge of the patient, to determine dosages and the best treatment for each individual patient. Neither the Publisher nor the author/editor/contributor (delete as appropriate) assumes any liability for any injury and/or damage to persons or property arising from this publication.

The Publisher

The publisher's policy is to use **paper manufactured from sustainable forests**

Printed in Spain

Contents

To our students,

past, present and future

Preface to the third edition

There is a world-wide shortage of anatomy teachers and there is also a significant and quite understandable reduction in dissecting room procedures, yet many branches of medicine and healthcare in general still require their students and practitioners to have a workable knowledge of anatomy. The portrayal of this anatomy by imaging methods has thus increased in importance over the last decade and now forms a significant proportion of the syllabus in many medical schools and anatomy courses. Many readers use this book in conjunction with atlases of anatomy as their first introduction to the human body and its interpretation in the studies of medicine, osteopathy and allied health sciences.

For this 3rd edition, we have upgraded considerable portions of the MR and CT areas of the chest, abdomen and pelvis to reflect the better resolution now available from modern scanners. Also, as a response to an extensive readers survey, some sections have been increased, others decreased and more line diagrams have been included to facilitate understanding of potentially difficult areas of interpretation, e.g. ultrasound. The general overall format has been maintained as it complements and supplements the McMinn Colour Atlas of Human Anatomy.

Our sincere thanks as always go to our co-authors, Drs Hourihan, Moore, Belli and Owen for their specialist contributions. Professor Gillian Needham has moved on to greater things in Medical Education and we thank her for her previous help. Richard Furn and Colin Arthur from Elsevier have been instrumental in the production of this 3rd edition and deserve full credit for their expertise.

The human body is still the same as it was 30,000 years ago; it is only our ability to see it and use this information in the study of medicine that keeps improving and changing direction. We hope that this new edition reflects these trends in modern medicine and will enable you, the reader, to understand the human body with greater clarity.

Jamie Weir, Peter Abrahams
May 2003

Acknowledgement for the 3rd edition

We would like to thank Dr Nicola H Strickland from the Hammersmith Hospital, London, and Dr Karen Duncan, from Aberdeen, for new images concerning the abdomen and fetal ultrasound respectively.

Preface to the second edition

In the four years since the production of the first edition of *An Imaging Atlas of Human Anatomy*, imaging has improved considerably, particularly in the fields of magnetic resonance and ultrasound. Over half the images have been updated for this new edition. Further improvements include the addition of completely new sections, limb ossification dates, line diagrams to improve the understanding of difficult areas and increased numbers of views where appropriate.

Most of the magnetic resonance images have been replaced with improved image recording, leading to greater clarity of anatomical detail. Ultrasound images have been similarly changed to be more comprehensive and cohesive. Examples of magnetic resonance angiography are included not only to demonstrate the remarkable beauty of these images but also to show the future of angiography into the next millennium.

It is with regret that one of our original authors, Professor Anne Hemingway, has left the team, but our thanks go to her for all her help and encouragement. We have pestered more outside contributors, as is evident from the list of acknowledgements, and our thanks go to them for their images and specialist expertise.

The CD-ROM version of our first edition was successfully launched late in 1995. The multimedia platform offers real-time ultrasound sequences, self-testing features and fully interactive labelling. Version 2.0 of the CD-ROM will be launched alongside this new edition of the book.

Imaging has opened up further anatomical areas to study and will continue to do so. We hope this new edition will stimulate its readers to explore the body through imaging as a key to its understanding.

Jamie Weir, Peter Abrahams
September 1996

Preface to the first edition

Imaging methods used to display normal human anatomy have improved dramatically over the last few decades. The ability to demonstrate the soft tissues by using the modern technologies of magnetic resonance imaging, X-ray computed tomography, and ultrasound has greatly facilitated our understanding of the link between anatomy as shown in the dissecting room and that necessary for clinical practice. This Atlas has been produced because of the new technology and the fundamental changes that are occurring in the teaching of anatomy. It enables the preclinical medical student to relate to basic anatomy while, at the same time, providing a comprehensive study guide for the clinical interpretation of imaging, applicable for all undergraduate and postgraduate levels.

Several distinguished authors, experts in their own fields of imaging, have contributed to this book, which has benefited from editorial integration to ensure balance and cohesion. The Atlas is designed to complement and supplement the *Colour Atlas of Human Anatomy* by McMinn.

Duplication of images occurs only where it is necessary to demonstrate anatomical points of interest or difficulty. Similarly, examples of different imaging modalities of the same anatomical region are only included if they contribute to a better understanding of the region shown. Radiographs that show important landmarks in limb ossification centre development, together with examples of some common congenital anomalies, are also documented. In certain sections, notably MR and CT, the legends may cover more than one page, so that a specific structure can be followed in continuity through various levels and planes.

Human anatomy does not alter, but our methods of demonstrating it have changed significantly. Modern imaging allows certain structures and their relationships to be seen for the first time, and this has aided us in their interpretation. Knowledge and understanding of radiological anatomy are fundamental to all those involved in patient care, from the nurse and the paramedic to medical students and clinicians.

Jamie Weir, Peter Abrahams
February 1992

guide to ossification tables

Ossification tables, such as the one shown on the right, appear throughout this book.

The key to these tables is as follows:
(c) = cartilage
(m) = membrane
miu = months of intrauterine life
wiu = weeks of intrauterine life
mths = months
yrs = years

And the rule to remember is: girls before boys.

CLAVICLE (m)	Appears	Fused
Lateral end	5 wiu	20+ yrs
Medial end	15 yrs	20+ yrs
SCAPULA (c)		
Body	8 wiu	15 yrs
Coracoid	<1 yr	20 yrs
Coracoid base	Puberty	15–20 yrs
Acromion	Puberty	15–20 yrs

Introduction

Access to the arterial system in order to produce an arteriogram (angiogram) is usually obtained by puncture and catheterisation of a femoral artery under local anaesthesia. Radiographic contrast medium is then injected into the vessel in the area under examination. If, for some reason, access via the femoral artery is not possible (owing to iliac occlusive disease or the presence of a graft, for example), alternative sites, such as the brachial or axillary artery, can be used. Translumbar aortography (TLA), a method of arteriography that involves direct percutaneous puncture of the aorta, is now less commonly employed as it does not allow selective catheterisation of aortic branches and hence percutaneous interventional vascular procedures cannot be performed. The development of new technology has meant that the aorta and the main upper and lower limb arteries can be visualised from an intravenous injection of contrast medium (into brachial vein, superior vena cava or right atrium), obviating the need for arterial puncture in some patients. This technique employs digital subtraction angiography (DSA), whereby unwanted background information is 'subtracted', leaving only an image of the blood vessels. Images of arteries obtained by injection into a vein are referred to as intravenous DSA examinations (IV DSA). DSA images of arteries can, of course, be obtained by direct intra-arterial injection (IA DSA).

Manual photographic subtraction of background information can also be performed with conventional (nondigital) arteriography. Subtraction, either photographic or digital, is used in cases in which fine vascular detail is required and can be simply recognised by the fact that, in contrast to an unsubtracted film, the arteries appear black as opposed to white. Different radiographic projections are sometimes employed to visualise best the vasculature; for example, in the aortic arch an anteroposterior view may not clearly show the origins of the vessels arising from the arch as they are very close to each other and may be superimposed. A left anterior oblique position opens the arch, allowing better visualisation of the origins of the brachiocephalic, left carotid and subclavian arteries. The angiograms in this book use the anteroposterior (AP) projection, unless otherwise indicated.

Veins may be visualised in the same way as the arteries, by direct puncture and catheterisation (via the femoral vein in most instances), for example. The veins of the upper and lower limbs are imaged by injecting contrast medium via an 18G or 20G needle placed in a peripheral vein, such as in the dorsum of the foot or hand, or the antecubital fossa. Alternatively, if imaging from an arterial injection is continued over a prolonged period of time, the arterial, capillary and venous phases can be recorded and venous anatomy visualised; this is a particularly useful way of visualising the portal venous system without necessitating direct trans-splenic or transhepatic puncture.

Specialist texts should be consulted for details of arterial puncture, catheterisation and imaging techniques and for information on the type of equipment used in angiography.

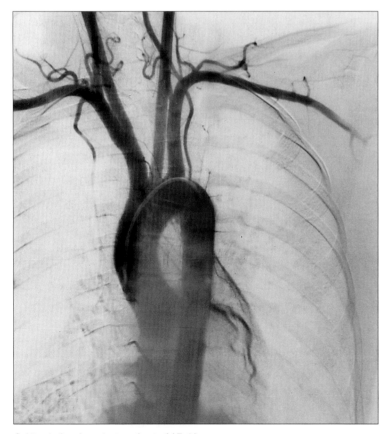

Subtracted arch aortogram (page 115, b).

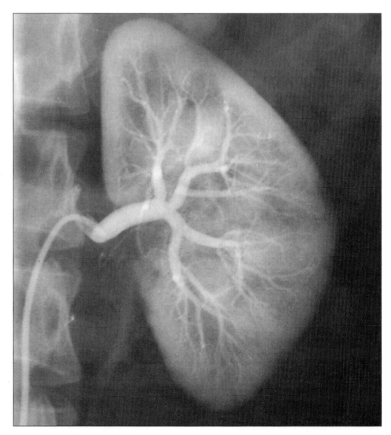

Renal arteriogram (page 150, a).

Computed tomography

The limitation of all plain radiographic techniques is the two dimensional representation of three dimensional structures: the linear attenuation co-efficient of all the tissues in the path of the x-ray beam form the image.

Computed tomography (CT) obtains a series of different angular x-ray projections that are processed by a computer to give a section of specified thickness. The CT image comprises a regular matrix of picture elements (pixels). All of the tissues contained within the pixel attenuate the x-ray projections and result in a mean attenuation value for the pixel. This value is compared with the attenuation value of water and is displayed on a scale (the Hounsfield Scale). Water is said to have an attenuation of 0 Hounsfield units (HU), and the scale is 2000HU wide. Air typically has an HU number of –1000; fat is approximately –100 HU; soft tissues are in the range +20 to +70HU; and bone is usually greater than +400HU.

Modern multislice helical CT scanners can obtain images in sub-second times and imaging of the whole body from the top of the head to the thighs can take as little as a single breath hold of 20 – 30 seconds. The fast scan times allow dynamic imaging of arteries and veins at different times after the injection of intravenous contrast agents. This technique is demonstrated in the new section on abdominal CT (pages 122-126), where the same patient is imaged during both the arterial and venous phases allowing the vascular anatomy to be shown to its full extent.

Digital images are stored on an archive and form part of an electronic storage record that is becoming common-place throughout the world, namely a PACS (Picture Archiving and Communication System). PACS allows interrogation of images via an electronic network so that those images (and reports) may be visualised at a distance, for example, on the wards or at another hospital. The Electronic Patient Record (EPR), where all patient information is stored, is developing rapidly and gaining acceptance allowing a marked improvement in data handling.

No specific preparation is required for CT examinations of the brain, spine or musculo-skeletal system. Studies of the chest, abdomen and pelvis usually require intravenous contrast medium that contains iodine, so enhancing the arteries and veins and defining their relationships to a greater extent. Opacification of the bowel in CT studies of the abdomen and pelvis can be accomplished by oral ingestion of a water soluble contrast medium from 24 hours prior to the examination to show the colon, combined with further oral intake 0 – 60 minutes, prior to the scan, for outlining the stomach and small bowel. Occasionally direct insertion of rectal contrast to show the distal large bowel may be required.

Generally all studies are performed with the patient supine and images are obtained in the transverse or axial plain. Modern CT scanners allow up to 25 degrees of gantry angulation, which is particularly valuable in spinal imaging. Occasionally, direct coronal images are obtained in the investigation of cranial and maxillo-facial abnormalities; in these cases the patient lies prone with the neck extended and the gantry appropriately angled.

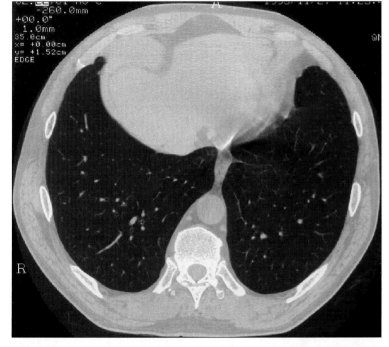

Lungs (page 99, n) axial CT image

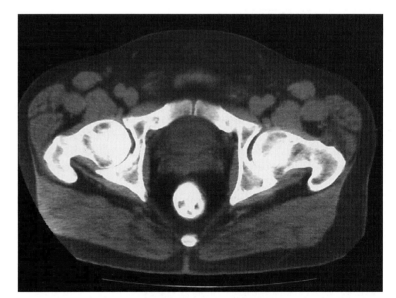

Male pelvis (page 158, c), axial CT image

Magnetic resonance imaging

Magnetic resonance imaging (MRI) combines a strong magnetic field and radiofrequency (RF) energy to study the distribution and behaviour of hydrogen protons in fat and water.

The spinning proton of the hydrogen nucleus can be thought of as a tiny bar magnet, with a north and south pole. In the absence of an external magnetic field, the magnetic moments of all of the protons in the body are randomly arranged. However, when the patient is placed in a strong magnetic field these magnetic moments align either with or against the field lines of the magnet. A small excess of magnetic moments align with the field, so that a net magnetic vector is established.

RF energy is used to generate a second magnetic field, perpendicular to the static magnetic field of the machine. The result of this second magnetic field is to rotate or 'flip' the protons away from the static magnetic field; the amount of rotation depends on the quantity of RF energy absorbed. Once the RF field is switched off, the protons experience only the effects of the static magnetic field and flip back to their original position. During this return to equilibrium, a process called 'relaxation', protons emit the RF energy they had acquired. This energy is detected by the antenna in the MRI machine, digitised, amplified and, finally, spatially encoded by the array processor. The resulting images are displayed on the operator's console and can be recorded on hard copy (for viewing) or transferred to magnetic tape or optical disc (for storage).

MRI systems are graded according to the strength of the magnetic field they produce. High-field systems are those capable of producing a magnetic field strength of 1–2 Tesla (T; 10 000–20 000 Gauss); mid-field systems operate at 0.35–0.5 T; and low-field systems produce a field strength of less than 0.2 T. Mid- and high-field systems use superconducting magnets in which the coils of copper wire are kept in a superconducting state (−269°C) by being immersed in an insulated helium bath. Electromagnets are fitted in resistive systems and are limited by heating factors to 0.35 T. Low-field systems use permanently magnetised metal cores, limiting field strength to around 0.2 T.

MRI does not present any recognised biological hazard. Patients who have any form of pacemaker or implanted electro-inductive device must not be examined. Other prohibited items include ferromagnetic intracranial aneurysm slips, certain types of cardiac valve replacement and intra-ocular metallic foreign bodies. Generally, it is safe to examine patients who have extracranial vascular clips and orthopaedic prostheses, but these may cause local artefacts. Loose metal items must be excluded from the examination room.

The preparation for an MR examination is simple. Patients wear metal-free clothes and must answer a rigorous safety questionnaire. Antiperistaltic agents (e.g. parenteral hyoscine N-butylbromide or glucagon) are often used in abdominal and pelvic examinations. Software techniques counteract respiratory motion for chest and abdominal imaging. Electrocardiographic gating is used in cardiac studies.

MR images may be obtained in any orthogonal or non-orthogonal plane. There is a wide range of pulse sequences, each of which provides a different image contrast. An intravenous injection of contrast medium (a gadolinium complex) may be given to enhance the visualisation of tumours, and inflammatory and vascular abnormalities.

Magnetic resonance angiography

The appearance of blood vessels depends on the pulse sequence used to produce images. With the spin echo technique, the time that elapses between exciting protons and receiving the return signal (the echo time) is such that excited blood has flowed out of the region; this volume of blood is replaced by unexcited blood which does not produce a signal, resulting in a flow void.

Gradient echo sequences use short echo-collection times and more frequent RF excitations, so that protons in stationary tissues do not fully relax, reducing the signal they generate. Protons entering the slice, however, are fully relaxed and thus produce a high signal (the 'time of flight effect'), so that blood vessels appear as bright structures against a dark background. Images can be displayed as three-dimensional MR angiograms, which can be viewed from any angle.

Another MR angiography technique uses additional magnetic fields to encode the phase of moving protons in blood vessels. A complete assessment of flow requires three acquisitions, each encoded by one of the three orthogonal gradients. These are summed to produce a 'phase contrast' MR angiogram. Phase differences can be quantified to provide estimates of flow velocity.

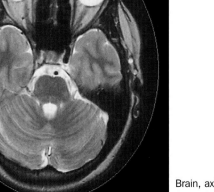

Brain, axial MR image
(page 34, b).

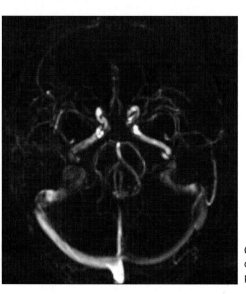

Circle of Willis MRA veins
of the brain, axial
projection (page 33, b).

Ultrasound

In contrast with the other images in this book, ultrasound images do not depend on the use of electromagnetic wave forms. It is the properties of high-frequency sound waves (longitudinal waves) and their interaction with biological tissues that go to form these 'echograms'.

A sound wave of appropriate frequency (diagnostic range 3.5–10 MHz) is produced by piezo-electric principles. Both the size and shape of the emitting crystal and its resonant frequency are important factors in determining the course of the sound beam within the tissues to be examined.

As the beam passes through tissues, two important effects determine image production: attenuation and reflection. Attenuation is caused by the loss of energy from the system, due to absorption and reflection, refraction and beam divergence out of the range of the receiver. The greater the attenuation of the sound beam through the tissues, the lower the resultant signal intensity received. Reflection of sound waves within the range of the receiver produces the image, the texture of which is dependent upon differences in acoustic impedance between different tissues. Ultrasound imaging systems are sensitive to the very small changes in acoustic impedance within soft tissue.

Through the application of these basic principles, sophisticated hardware has been developed that converts the pulse–echo system, briefly described above, into a real-time two-dimensional sectional image. The addition of the facility to measure blood flow and velocity ultrasonically (using the Doppler principle) has led to the development and wide availability of duplex scanners.

The effects of shadowing and enhancement within an ultrasound image are of paramount importance. Systems are designed assuming an average attenuation through a depth of tissue, and are balanced to give an even intensity of signal for deep and superficial tissues. An acoustic shadow occurs when a tissue within the measured depth has a higher-than-average attenuation; all tissues deep to this will appear with a falsely lower intensity (shadowed). Conversely, a tissue with a lower-than-average attenuation will cause all tissues deep to it to appear falsely high in intensity (enhanced). Fibrous tissue, calcification and gas all produce acoustic shadows, whereas fluid-filled structures often cause enhancement.

If a selection of ultrasound transducers with varying frequencies, focusing mechanisms and shapes and sizes is available, visualisation of a wide range of tissues—from the neonatal brain to the soft tissues of the hand—becomes possible. Only relevant ultrasound images have been included in the book to illustrate a particular point or area, as the real-time nature of ultrasound precludes further coverage. Interpretation of the anatomy from static ultrasound images is more difficult than that from other imaging modalities because the technique is highly operator-dependent and provides information on tissue structure and form different from that of other imaging techniques.

1 Head, neck and brain

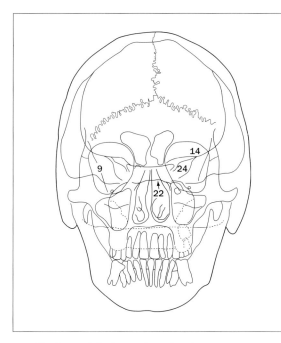

(a) Skull, occipitofrontal projection.
(b) Skull, demonstrating the foramina rotunda, occipitofrontal projection.

1 Basi-occiput
2 Body of sphenoid
3 Crista galli
4 Ethmoidal air cells
5 Floor of maxillary sinus (antrum)
6 Floor of pituitary fossa
7 Foramen rotundum
8 Frontal sinus
9 Greater wing of sphenoid
10 Inferior turbinate
11 Internal acoustic meatus
12 Lambdoid suture
13 Lateral mass of atlas (first cervical vertebra)
14 Lesser wing of sphenoid
15 Mastoid process
16 Middle turbinate
17 Nasal septum
18 Odontoid process (dens) of axis
   (second cervical vertebra)
19 Petrous part of temporal bone
20 Ramus of mandible
21 Sagittal suture
22 Sella turcica
23 Sphenoid air sinus
24 Superior orbital fissure
25 Temporal surface of greater wing of sphenoid

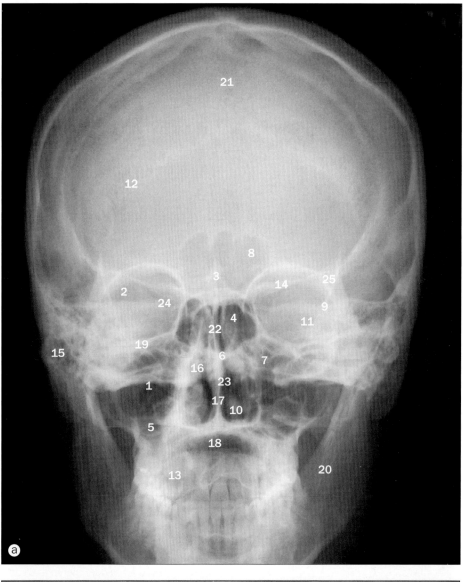

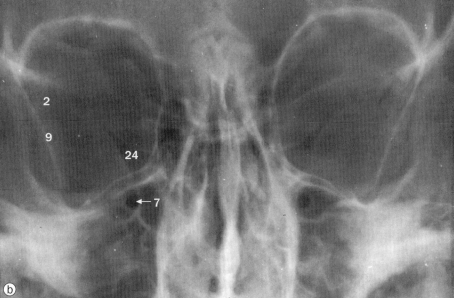

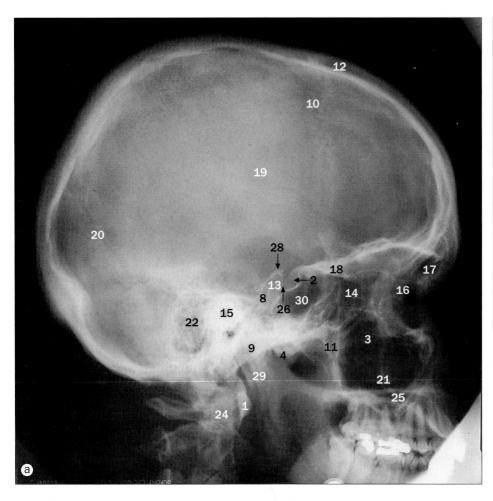

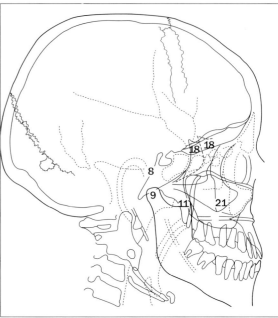

(a) Skull, lateral projection.

Pituitary fossa (sella turcica), (b) of a 7-year-old child, (c) of a 23-year-old woman, lateral projections.

1 Anterior arch of atlas (first cervical vertebra)	**11** Coronoid process of mandible	**22** Mastoid air cells
2 Anterior clinoid process	**12** Diploë	**23** Middle clinoid process
3 Arch of zygoma	**13** Dorsum sellae	**24** Odontoid process (dens) of axis
4 Articular tubercle for temporomandibular joint	**14** Ethmoidal air cells	(second cervical vertebra)
	15 External acoustic meatus	**25** Palatine process of maxilla
5 Basilar part of occipital bone	**16** Frontal process of zygoma	**26** Pituitary fossa (sella turcica)
6 Basisphenoid/basi-occiput synchondrosis	**17** Frontal sinus	**27** Planum sphenoidale
7 Carotid sulcus	**18** Greater wing of sphenoid	**28** Posterior clinoid process
8 Clivus	**19** Grooves for middle meningeal vessels	**29** Ramus of mandible
9 Condyle of mandible	**20** Lambdoid suture	**30** Sphenoidal sinus
10 Coronal suture	**21** Malar process of maxilla	**31** Tuberculum sellae

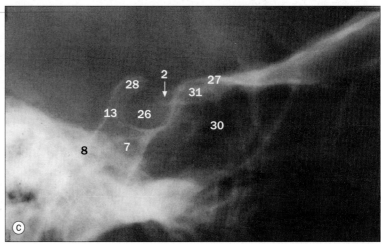

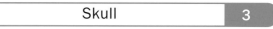

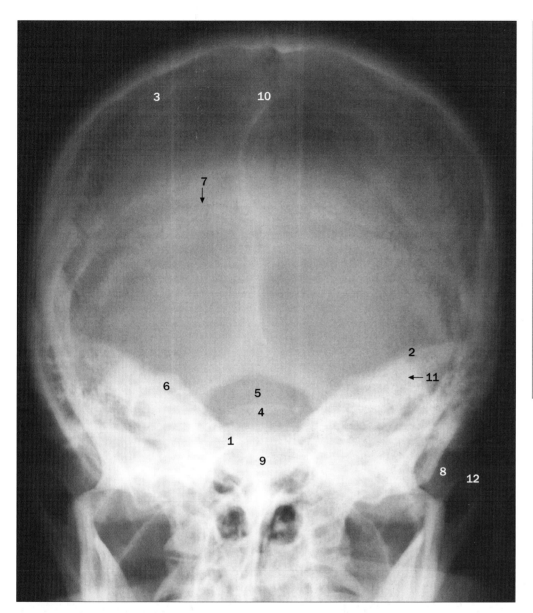

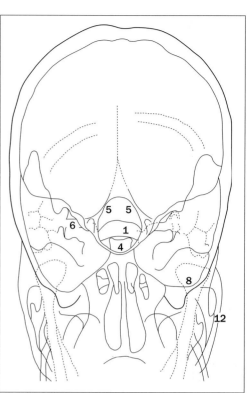

Skull, 30° fronto-occipital (Townes') projection.

1 Arch of atlas (first cervical vertebra)
2 Arcuate eminence of temporal bone
3 Coronal suture
4 Dorsum sellae
5 Foramen magnum
6 Internal acoustic meatus
7 Lambdoid suture
8 Mandibular condyle
9 Odontoid process (dens) of axis (second cervical vertebra)
10 Sagittal suture
11 Superior semicircular canal
12 Zygomatic arch

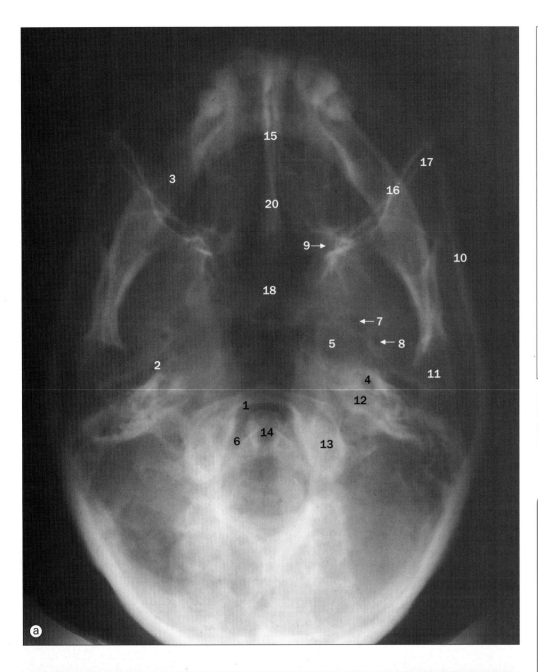

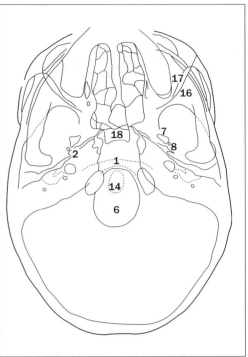

(a) Skull, submentovertical projection.
(b) Skull, with additional angulation for zygomatic arches, submentovertical projection.

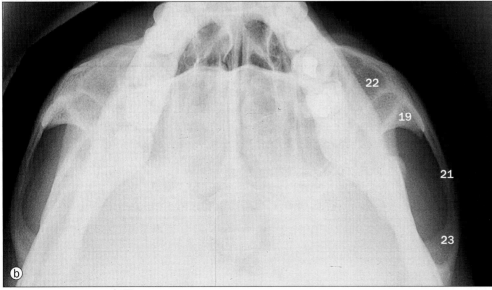

1 Anterior arch of atlas (first cervical vertebra)
2 Auditory (Eustachian) tube
3 Body of mandible
4 Carotid canal
5 Foramen lacerum
6 Foramen magnum
7 Foramen ovale
8 Foramen spinosum
9 Greater palatine foramen
10 Greater wing of sphenoid
11 Head of mandible
12 Jugular foramen
13 Occipital condyle
14 Odontoid process (dens) of axis (second cervical vertebra)
15 Perpendicular plate of ethmoid
16 Posterior margin of orbit
17 Posterior wall of maxillary sinus (antrum)
18 Sphenoidal sinus
19 Temporal process of zygomatic bone
20 Vomer
21 Zygomatic arch
22 Zygomatic bone
23 Zygomatic process of temporal bone

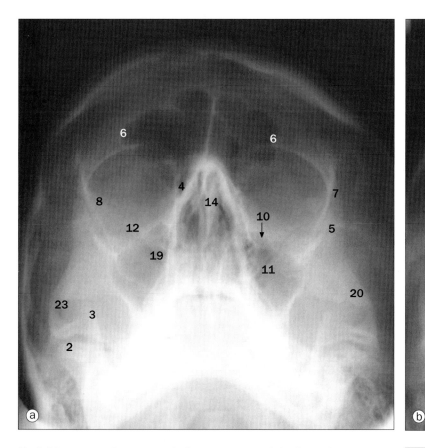

Facial bones and paranasal sinuses, (a) occipitofrontal projection, (b) occipitomental projection, (c) lateral projection.

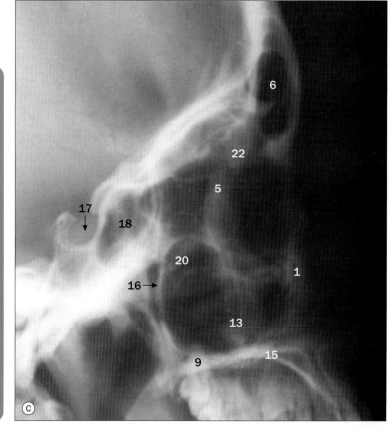

1	Anterior wall of maxillary sinus (antrum)
2	Condyle of mandible
3	Coronoid process of mandible
4	Ethmoidal sinuses
5	Frontal process of zygomatic bone
6	Frontal sinuses
7	Frontozygomatic suture
8	Greater wing of sphenoid
9	Horizontal plate of palatine bone
10	Infra-orbital foramen
11	Left maxillary sinus (antrum)
12	Lesser wing of sphenoid
13	Malar process of maxilla
14	Nasal septum
15	Palatine process of maxilla
16	Posterior wall of maxillary sinus (antrum)
17	Sella turcica
18	Sphenoidal sinus
19	Superior orbital fissure
20	Temporal process of zygomatic bone
21	Zygomatic arch
22	Zygomatic process of frontal bone
23	Zygomatic process of temporal bone

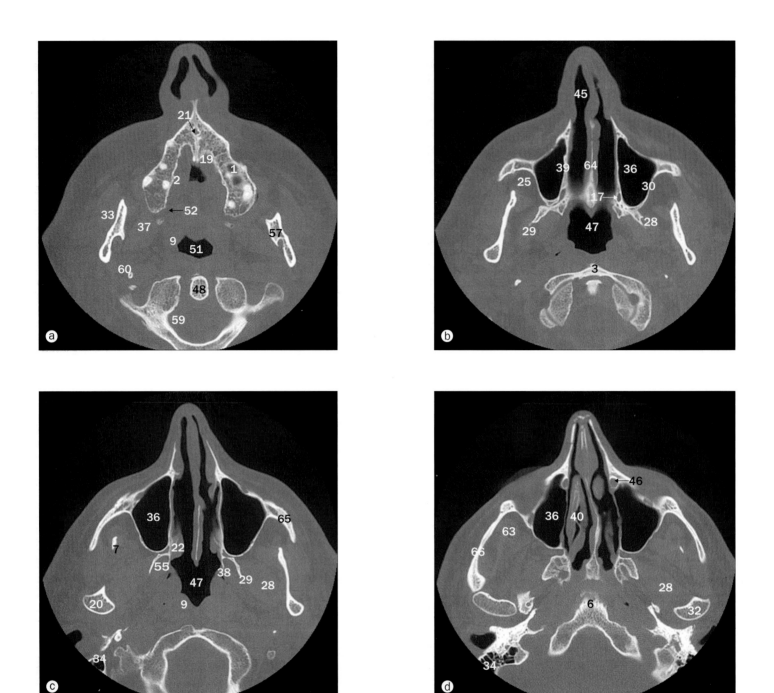

Facial bones and paranasal sinuses, axial CT images are demonstrated at the following levels: (a) alveolar process of the maxilla; (b) maxillary sinus; (c) arch of the atlas (C2); (d) zygomatic arch; (e) base of the skull; (f) sphenoid sinus; (g) ethmoidal sinuses; (h) optic nerve

1 Alveolar recess	**12** Foramen ovale	**24** Inferolateral recess
2 Alveolar rim	**13** Foramen spinosum	**25** Infratemporal fossa
3 Anterior arch of atlas (first cervical vertebra)	**14** Frontal bone	**26** Internal acoustic meatus
	15 Frontal sinus	**27** Lacrimal bone
4 Anterior clinoid process	**16** Globe	**28** Lateral pterygoid muscle
5 Anterior ethmoidal air cells	**17** Greater palatine canal	**29** Lateral pterygoid plate
6 Clivus	**18** Greater wing of sphenoid	**30** Lateral wall of maxillary sinus (antrum)
7 Coronoid process of mandible	**19** Hard palate	**31** Lens
8 Crista galli	**20** Head of mandible	**32** Mandibular condyle
9 Deglutitional muscles	**21** Incisive canal	**33** Masseter muscle
10 Dorsum sellae	**22** Inferior nasal concha (turbinate)	**34** Mastoid air cells
11 External acoustic canal	**23** Inferior orbital fissure	**35** Mastoid process

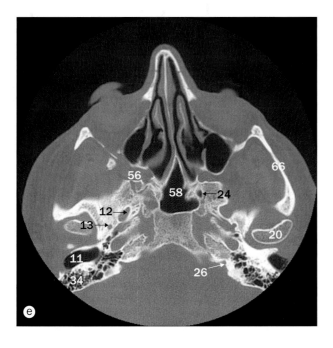

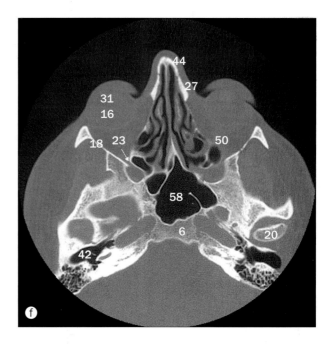

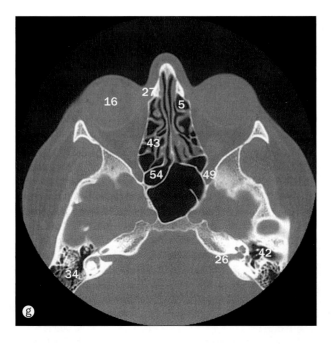

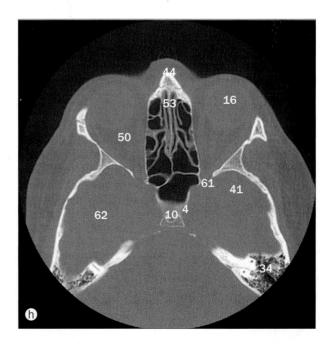

36	Maxillary sinus (antrum)	47	Nasopharynx	58	Sphenoidal sinus
37	Medial pterygoid muscle	48	Odontoid process (dens)	59	Spinal canal
38	Medial pterygoid plate	49	Optic canal	60	Styloid process
39	Medial wall of maxillary sinus (antrum)	50	Optic nerve	61	Superior orbital fissure
40	Middle concha (turbinate)	51	Oropharynx	62	Temporal lobe
41	Middle cranial fossa	52	Parapharyngeal space	63	Temporalis muscle
42	Middle ear cavity	53	Perpendicular plate of ethmoid bone	64	Vomer
43	Middle ethmoidal air cells	54	Posterior ethmoidal air cells	65	Zygoma
44	Nasal bone	55	Pterygoid fossa	66	Zygomatic arch
45	Nasal cavity	56	Pterygomaxillary fissure		
46	Nasolacrimal duct	57	Ramus of mandible		

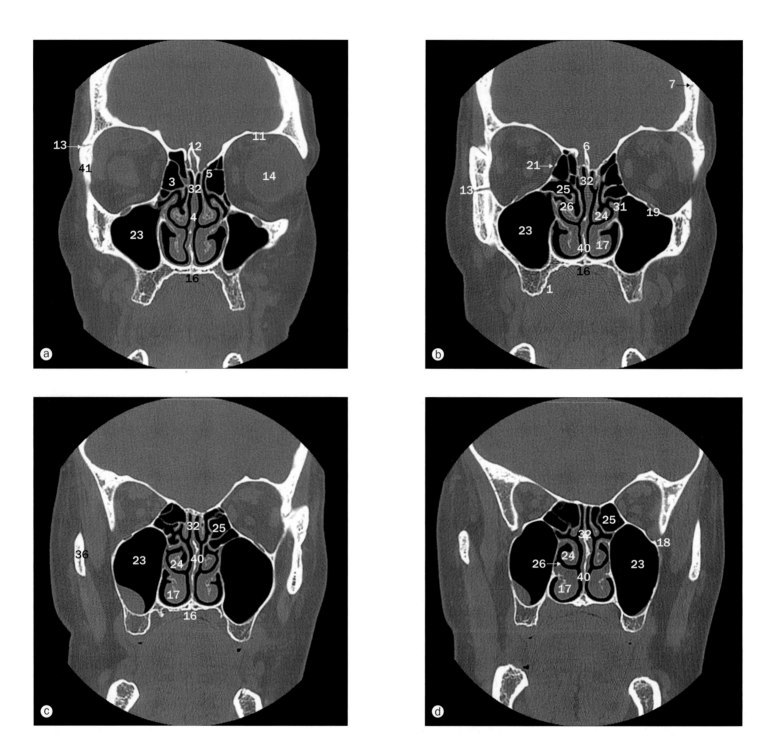

Facial bones and paranasal sinuses, coronal CT images are demonstrated at the following levels: (a) anterior ethmoidal sinuses; (b) optic nerve; (c) middle ethmoidal sinus and maxillary sinus; (d) posterior ethmoidal sinus; (e) posterior maxillary sinus; (f) anterior sphenoidal sinus; (g) middle sphenoidal sinus; (h) posterior sphenoidal sinus.

1	Alveolar rim	11	Frontal bone
2	Anterior clinoid process	12	Frontal sinus
3	Anterior ethmoidal air cells	13	Frontozygomatic suture
4	Cartilaginous portion of nasal septum	14	Globe
5	Cribriform plate	15	Greater wing of sphenoid
6	Crista galli	16	Hard palate
7	Diploë	17	Inferior nasal concha (turbinate)
8	Dorsum sellae	18	Inferior orbital fissure
9	Foramen lacerum	19	Infra-orbital canal
10	Foramen ovale	20	Infratemporal fossa

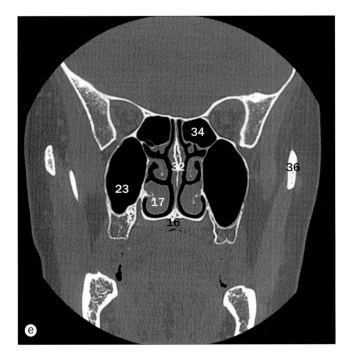

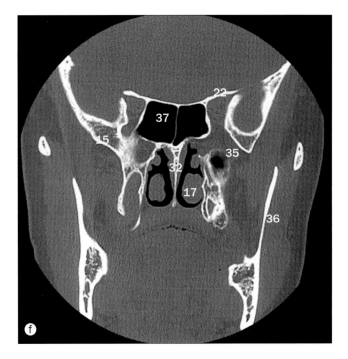

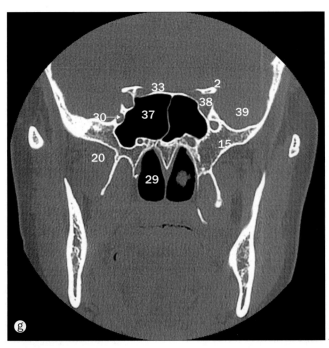

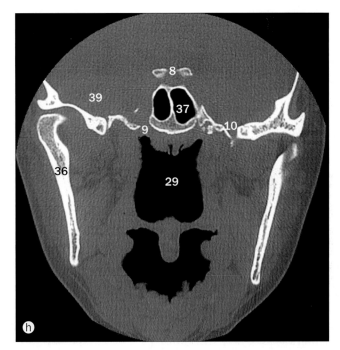

21	Lamina papyracea	
22	Lesser wing of sphenoid	
23	Maxillary sinus (antrum)	
24	Middle concha (turbinate)	
25	Middle ethmoidal air cells	
26	Middle meatus	
27	Nasal bone	
28	Nasolacrimal duct	
29	Nasopharynx	
30	Optic canal	
31	Ostium of antrum	

32	Perpendicular plate of ethmoidal bone
33	Planum sphenoidale
34	Posterior ethmoidal air cells
35	Pterygopalatine fossa
36	Ramus of mandible
37	Sphenoidal sinus
38	Superior orbital fissure
39	Temporal lobe
40	Vomer
41	Zygoma

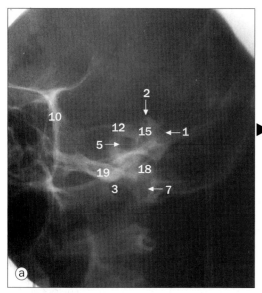

(a) Petrous temporal bone, postero-anterior oblique projection.

1 Aditus to mastoid antrum
2 Arcuate eminence of temporal bone
3 External acoustic meatus
4 Helix of pinna of ear
5 Internal acoustic meatus
6 Lateral sinus
7 Mandibular condyle
8 Mandibular fossa
9 Mastoid air cells
10 Orbital margin
11 Ossicles (malleus, incus)
12 Petrous part of temporal bone
13 Pinna of ear
14 Styloid process
15 Superior semicircular canal
16 Temporomandibular joint
17 Tip of mastoid process
18 Vestibular part of inner ear
19 Zygomatic arch

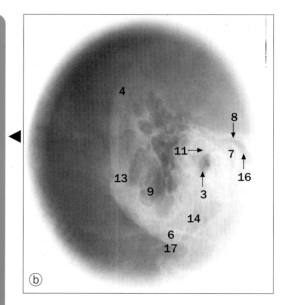

(b) Mastoid process, lateral oblique projection.

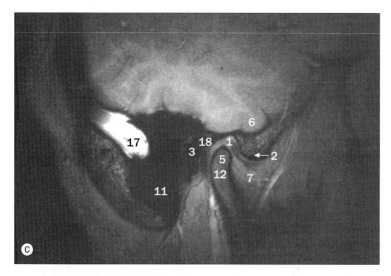

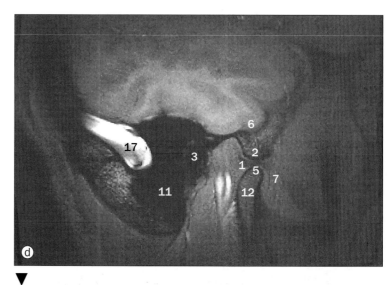

Temporomandibular joint, sagittal MR images, (c) closed, (d) open.
Radiographs of the temporomandibular joint, (e) closed, (f) open.

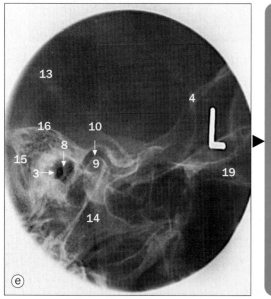

1 Articular disc
2 Articular tubercle of temporal bone
3 External acoustic meatus
4 Greater wing of sphenoid
5 Head of mandible
6 Inferior temporal gyrus
7 Lateral pterygoid muscle
8 Malleus
9 Mandibular condyle
10 Mandibular fossa
11 Mastoid process of temporal bone
12 Neck of mandible
13 Pinna of ear
14 Posterior border of ramus of mandible
15 Sinus plate
16 Tegmen tympani
17 Transverse sinus
18 Tympanic part of temporal bone
19 Zygomatic process of temporal bone

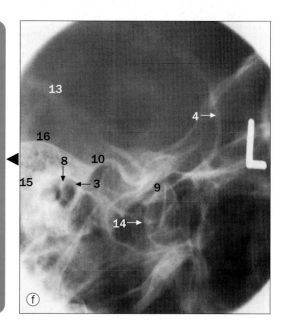

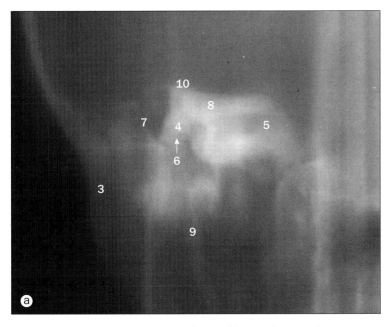

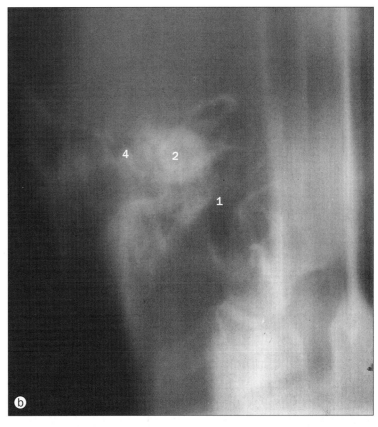

(a) Temporal bone, tomogram at level of internal acoustic meatus.

1	Carotid canal	7	Mastoid antrum
2	Cochlea	8	Petrous part of temporal
3	External acoustic meatus		bone
4	Incus	9	Styloid process of temporal
5	Internal acoustic meatus		bone
6	Malleus	10	Superior semicircular canal

(b) Temporal bone, tomogram at level of cochlea (image taken several millimetres anterior to section shown in (a)).

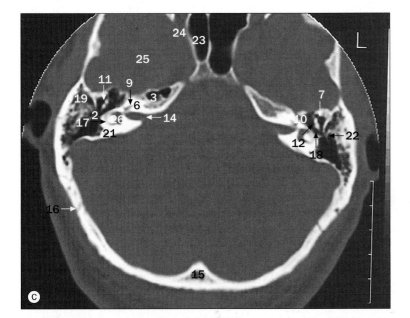

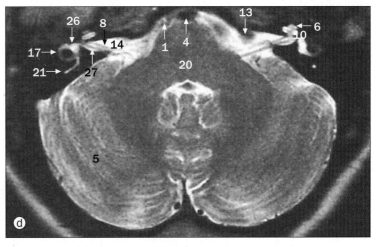

(c) Temporal bone, CT image.
(d) Temporal bone, axial MR image through cerebellopontine angle.

1	Abducens nerve	10	Geniculate ganglion	19	Mastoid air cells
2	Aditus ad antrum	11	Incudomalleolar joint	20	Pons
3	Aerated petrous apex	12	Incus	21	Posterior semicircular canal
4	Basilar artery in prepontine cistern	13	Inferior petrosal sinus	22	Scutum
5	Cerebellar hemisphere	14	Internal acoustic canal	23	Sphenoidal sinus
6	Cochlea	15	Internal occipital protuberance	24	Superior orbital fissure
7	Epitympanum	16	Lambdoid suture	25	Temporal lobe
8	Facial nerve	17	Lateral semicircular canal	26	Vestibule
9	Facial nerve (first part)	18	Malleus	27	Vestibulocochlear nerve

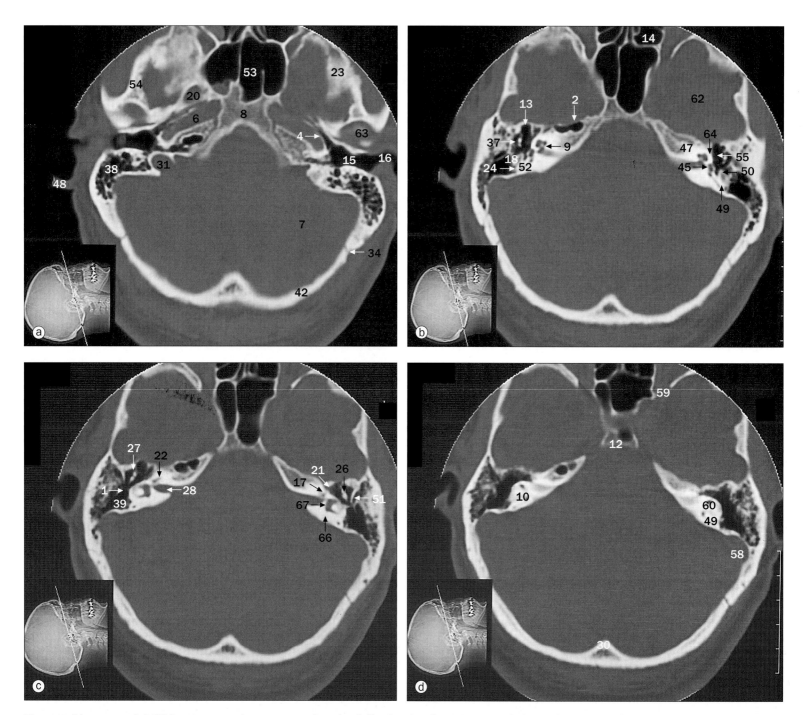

Temporal bones, axial CT images are demonstrated at the following levels: (**a**) external acoustic canal; (**b**) cochlea; (**c**) internal acoustic canal and vestibule; (**d**) upper middle ear and mastoid.

1 Aditus to antrum	**12** Dorsum sellae	**23** Greater wing of sphenoid
2 Aeration of petrous apex	**13** Epitympanic space	**24** Horizontal portion of canal for facial nerve
3 Atlanto-occipital joint	**14** Ethmoidal air cells	**25** Hypoglossal canal
4 Auditory (Eustachian) tube	**15** External acoustic canal	**26** Incudomalleolar joint
5 Brainstem	**16** External acoustic meatus	**27** Incus
6 Carotid canal	**17** Facial nerve (first part)	**28** Internal acoustic canal
7 Cerebellum	**18** Facial recess	**29** Internal acoustic meatus
8 Clivus	**19** Falciform crest	**30** Internal occipital protuberance
9 Cochlea	**20** Foramen ovale	**31** Jugular foramen
10 Cochlear aqueduct	**21** Geniculate ganglion	**32** Jugular fossa
11 Descending segment of facial nerve	**22** Greater petrosal nerve	**33** Jugular tubercle

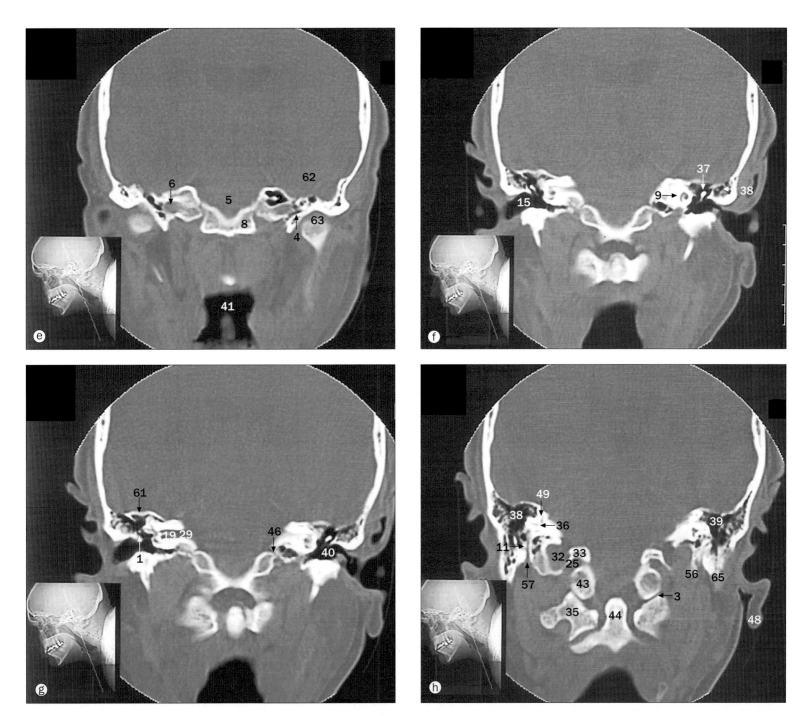

Temporal bones, coronal CT images are demonstrated at the following levels:
(e) posterior temporomandibular joint; (f) external acoustic meatus and vestibule; (g) internal acoustic meatus; (h) mastoid.

34 Lambdoid suture	**45** Oval window	**57** Stylomastoid foramen
35 Lateral mass of atlas (first cervical vertebra)	**46** Petro-occipital fissure	**58** Sulcus of sigmoid venous sinus
36 Lateral semicircular canal	**47** Petrous temporal bone	**59** Superior orbital fissure
37 Malleus	**48** Pinna of ear	**60** Superior semicircular canal
38 Mastoid air cells	**49** Posterior semicircular canal	**61** Tegmen tympani
39 Mastoid antrum	**50** Pyramidal eminence	**62** Temporal lobe
40 Middle ear cavity	**51** Scutum	**63** Temporomandibular joint
41 Nasopharynx	**52** Sinus tympani	**64** Tensor tympani muscle
42 Occipital bone	**53** Sphenoidal sinus	**65** Tip of mastoid process
43 Occipital condyle	**54** Squamous temporal bone	**66** Vestibular aqueduct
44 Odontoid process (dens)	**55** Stapes	**67** Vestibule
	56 Styloid process	

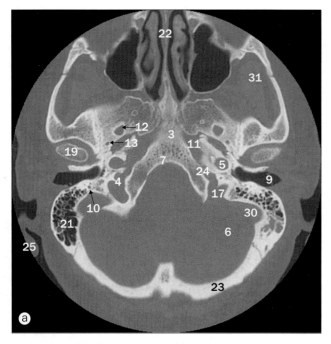
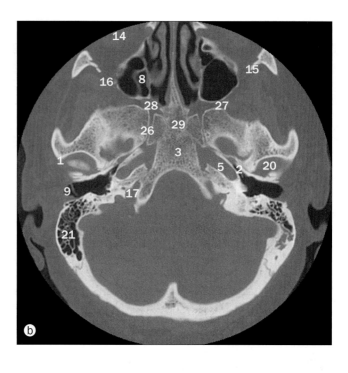

(a) and (b) Skull base, axial CT images.

1 Articular condyle	**12** Foramen ovale	**23** Occipital bone
2 Auditory (Eustachian) tube	**13** Foramen spinosum	**24** Petro-occipital fissure
3 Basisphenoid	**14** Globe	**25** Pinna of ear
4 Caroticojugular spine	**15** Greater wing of sphenoid	**26** Pterygoid (vidian) canal
5 Carotid canal	**16** Inferior orbital fissure	**27** Pterygomaxillary fissure
6 Cerebellar hemisphere	**17** Jugular foramen	**28** Pterygopalantine fossa
7 Clivus	**18** Lens	**29** Sphenoidal sinus
8 Ethmoidal air cells	**19** Mandibular condyle	**30** Sulcus of sigmoid venous sinus
9 External acoustic meatus	**20** Mandibular fossa	**31** Temporalis muscle
10 Facial nerve canal	**21** Mastoid air cells	
11 Foramen lacerum	**22** Nasal septum	

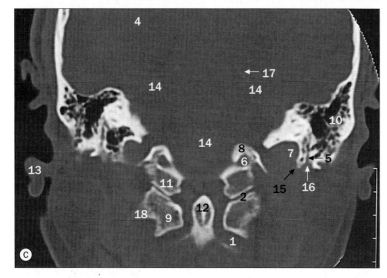
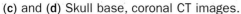

(c) and (d) Skull base, coronal CT images.

1 Atlanto-axial joint	**7** Jugular fossa	**13** Pinna of ear
2 Atlanto-occipital joint	**8** Jugular tubercle	**14** Posterior fossa
3 Axis (second cervical vertebra)	**9** Lateral mass of atlas (first cervical vertebra)	**15** Styloid process
4 Cerebral hemisphere	**10** Mastoid air cells	**16** Stylomastoid foramen
5 Descending segment of canal for facial nerve	**11** Occipital condyle	**17** Tentorium cerebelli
6 Hypoglossal canal	**12** Odontoid process (dens)	**18** Transverse process of atlas

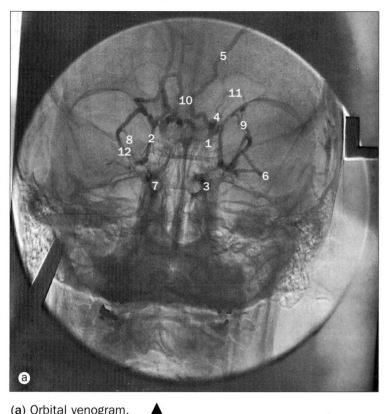

(a) Orbital venogram. ▲

1 Angular veins
2 Anterior collateral vein
3 Cavernous sinus
4 First part of superior ophthalmic vein
5 Frontal veins
6 Inferior ophthalmic vein
7 Internal carotid artery
8 Medial collateral vein
9 Second part of superior ophthalmic vein
10 Superficial connecting vein
11 Supraorbital vein
12 Third part of superior ophthalmic vein

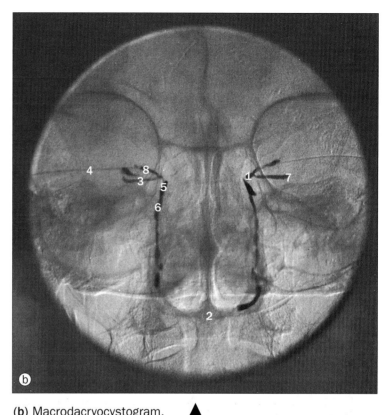

(b) Macrodacryocystogram. ▲

1 Common canaliculus	5 Lacrimal sac
2 Hard palate	6 Nasolacrimal duct
3 Inferior canaliculus	7 Site of lacrimal punctum
4 Lacrimal catheters	8 Superior canaliculus

(c) Globe, axial MR image.

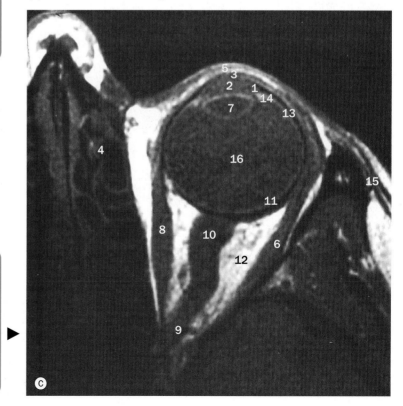

1 Anterior chamber	10 Optic nerve
2 Aqueous humour	11 Retina and choroid
3 Cornea	12 Retro-orbital fat
4 Ethmoidal sinuses	13 Sclera
5 Eyelid	14 Suspensory ligament
6 Lateral rectus muscle	of the lens
7 Lens	15 Temporalis muscle
8 Medial rectus muscle	16 Vitreous
9 Ophthalmic artery	

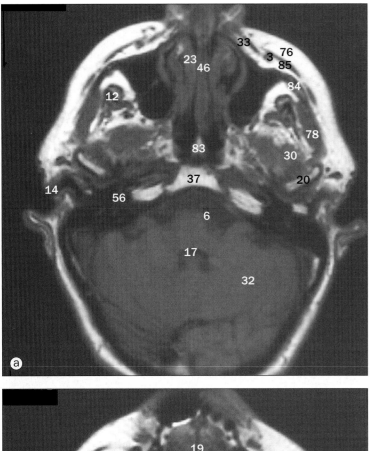

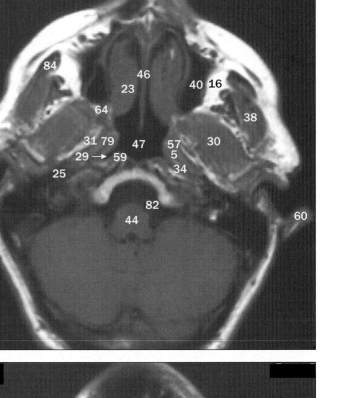

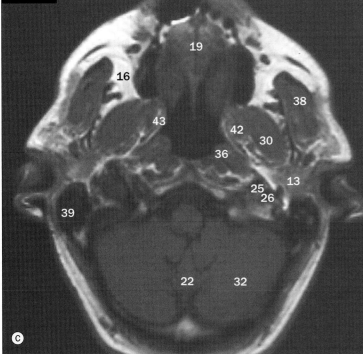

(a)–(h) Nasopharynx and oropharynx, axial MR images.

1 Alveolar process of maxilla	**8** Body of mandible	**16** Fat in infratemporal fossa	**25** Internal carotid artery
2 Anterior arch of atlas (first cervical vertebra)	**9** Buccinator muscle	**17** Fourth ventricle	**26** Internal jugular vein
3 Anterior facial vein	**10** Cerebellar tonsils	**18** Genioglossus muscle	**27** Intrinsic muscles of tongue
4 Ascending pharyngeal artery	**11** Cerebrospinal fluid in subarachnoid space	**19** Hard palate	**28** Lateral mass of atlas (first cervical vertebra)
5 Auditory (Eustachian) tube	**12** Coronoid process of mandible	**20** Head of mandible	**29** Lateral pharyngeal recess
6 Basilar artery	**13** Deep lobe of parotid gland	**21** Hyoglossus muscle	**30** Lateral pterygoid muscle
7 Body of axis (second cervical vertebra)	**14** External acoustic canal	**22** Inferior cerebellar vermis	**31** Lateral pterygoid plate
	15 External carotid artery	**23** Inferior nasal concha	**32** Left cerebellar hemisphere
		24 Inferior oblique muscle	

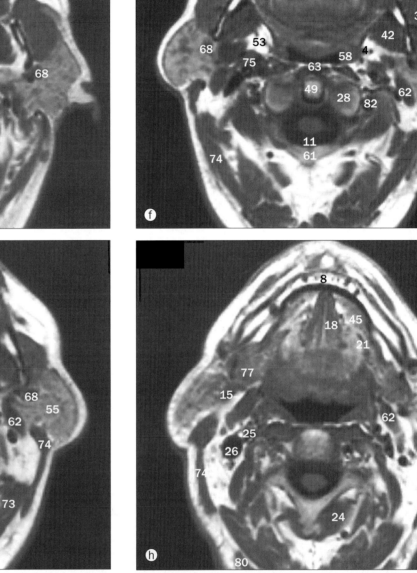

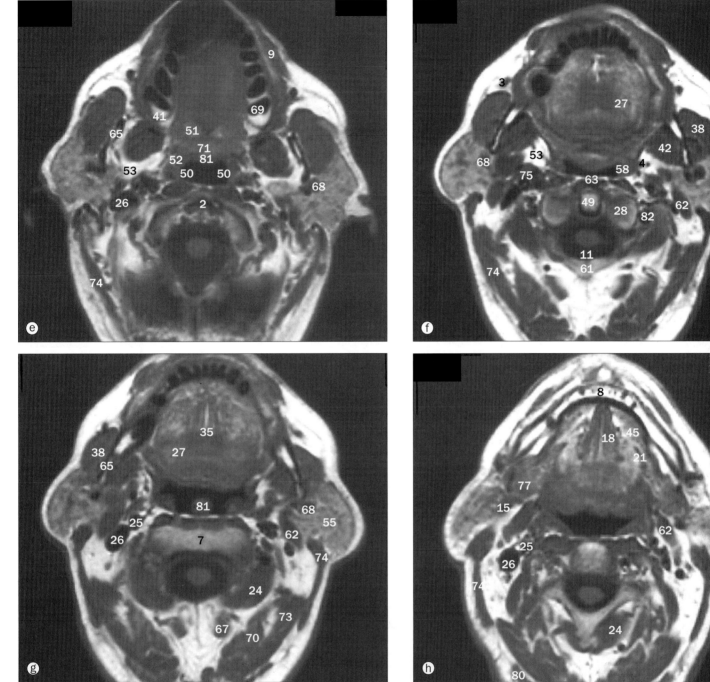

33	Levator labii superioris alaeque nasi muscle	47	Nasopharynx	59	Pharyngobasilar fascia	73	Splenius capitis muscle
34	Levator veli palatini muscle	48	Occipital condyle	60	Pinna of ear	74	Sternocleidomastoid muscle
35	Lingual septum	49	Odontoid process (dens)	61	Posterior arch of atlas	75	Stylopharyngeus muscle
36	Longus capitis muscle	50	Oropharynx	62	Posterior belly of digastric muscle	76	Subcutaneous fat
37	Marrow of clivus	51	Palatine tonsils			77	Submandibular gland
38	Masseter muscle	52	Palatopharyngeus muscle	63	Posterior pharyngeal wall	78	Temporalis muscle
39	Mastoid process	53	Parapharyngeal space	64	Pterygomaxillary fissure	79	Tensor veli palatini muscle
40	Maxillary sinus (antrum)	54	Parotid duct	65	Ramus of mandible	80	Trapezius muscle
41	Maxillary tuberosity	55	Parotid gland	66	Rectus capitis anterior muscle	81	Uvula
42	Medial pterygoid muscle	56	Petrous portion of temporal bone	67	Rectus capitis muscle	82	Vertebral artery
43	Medial pterygoid plate			68	Retromandibular vein	83	Vomer
44	Medulla oblongata	57	Pharyngeal cartilaginous end of auditory tube (torus tubarius)	69	Root of upper molar tooth	84	Zygomatic arch
45	Mylohyoid muscle			70	Semispinalis capitis muscle	85	Zygomaticus muscle
46	Nasal septal cartilage	58	Pharyngeal constrictor muscle	71	Soft palate		
				72	Spinal cord		

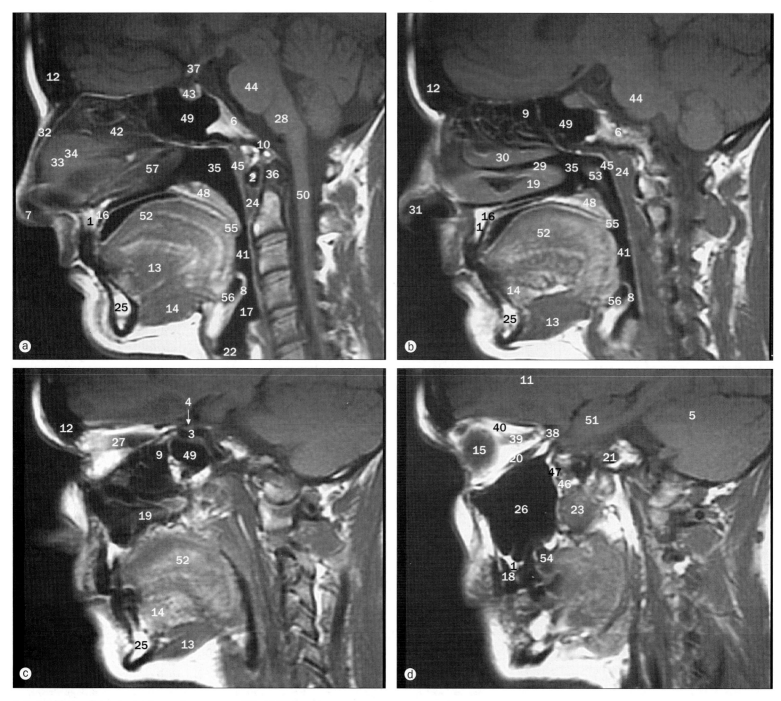

(a)–(d) Nasopharynx and oropharynx, sagittal MR images.

1 Alveolar process of maxilla	14 Geniohyoid muscle	29 Middle meatus	43 Pituitary gland
2 Anterior arch of atlas (first cervical vertebra)	15 Globe	30 Middle nasal concha	44 Pons
3 Cavernous portion of internal carotid artery	16 Hard palate	31 Nasal ala	45 Posterior wall of pharynx
	17 Hypopharynx	32 Nasal bone	46 Pterygomaxillary fissure
4 Cavernous sinus	18 Incisor tooth	33 Nasal septal cartilage	47 Pterygopalatine fossa
5 Cerebellar hemisphere	19 Inferior nasal concha	34 Nasal septum	48 Soft palate
6 Clivus	20 Inferior rectus muscle	35 Nasopharynx	49 Sphenoidal sinus
7 Columella	21 Internal carotid artery	36 Odontoid process (dens)	50 Spinal cord
8 Epiglottis	22 Larynx	37 Optic chiasma	51 Temporal lobe
9 Ethmoidal air cells	23 Lateral pterygoid muscle	38 Optic foramen	52 Tongue
10 Foramen magnum	24 Longus capitis muscle	39 Optic nerve	53 Torus tubarius
11 Frontal lobe	25 Mandible	40 Orbital fat	54 Upper molar tooth
12 Frontal sinus	26 Maxillary sinus (antrum)	41 Oropharynx	55 Uvula
13 Genioglossus muscle	27 Medial rectus muscle	42 Perpendicular plate of ethmoid bone	56 Vallecula
	28 Medulla oblongata		57 Vomer

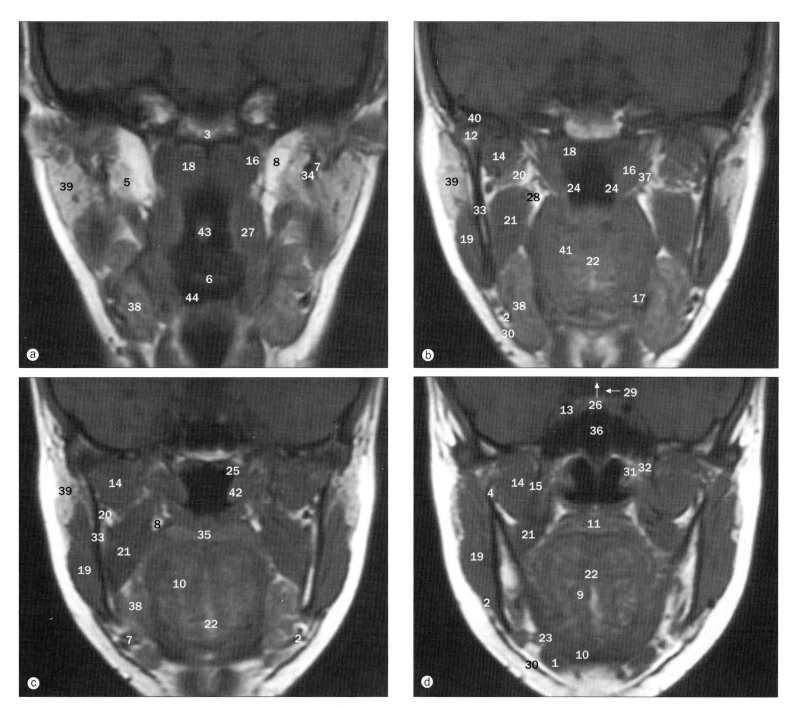

(a)–(d) Nasopharynx and oropharynx, coronal MR images.

1 Anterior belly of digastric muscle	12 Head of mandible	23 Mylohyoid muscle	34 Retromandibular vein
2 Anterior facial vein	13 Internal carotid artery	24 Nasopharynx	35 Soft palate
3 Clivus	14 Lateral pterygoid muscle	25 Opening of auditory (Eustachian) tube	36 Sphenoidal sinus
4 Coronoid process of mandible	15 Lateral pterygoid plate	26 Optic chiasma	37 Stylopharyngeus muscle
5 Deep lobe of parotid gland	16 Levator veli palatini muscle and tensor veli palatini muscle	27 Palatal constrictor muscles	38 Submandibular gland
6 Epiglottis	17 Lingual artery	28 Palatine artery	39 Superficial lobe of parotid gland
7 Facial artery	18 Longus capitis muscle	29 Pituitary stalk	40 Temporomandibular joint
8 Fat in parapharyngeal space	19 Masseter muscle	30 Platysma muscle	41 Tongue
9 Genioglossus muscle	20 Maxillary artery	31 Pterygoid (vidian) canal	42 Torus tubarius
10 Geniohyoid muscle	21 Medial pterygoid muscle	32 Pterygoid process of sphenoid	43 Uvula
11 Hard palate	22 Median raphe of tongue	33 Ramus of mandible	44 Vallecula

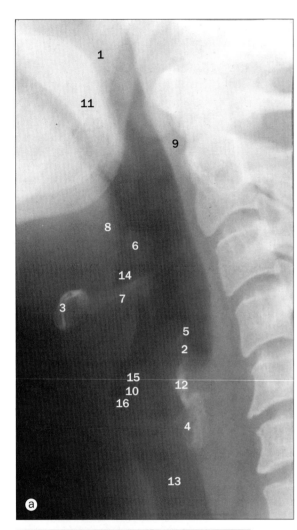

(a) Soft tissues of the neck, lateral projection. ◄

1 Air in nasopharynx	9 Retropharyngeal soft tissues
2 Arytenoid cartilage	10 Sinus of larynx
3 Body of hyoid bone	11 Soft palate
4 Cricoid cartilage	12 Superior horn of thyroid cartilage
5 Cuneiform cartilage	13 Trachea
6 Epiglottis	14 Vallecula
7 Greater horn of hyoid bone	15 Vestibular fold
8 Posterior aspect of tongue	16 Vocal fold

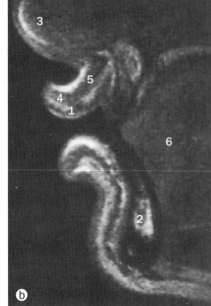

(b) The kiss, sagittal MR image.

1 Deltoid insertion of levator muscle
2 Mandible
3 Nose
4 Pars marginalis of orbicularis oris muscle
5 Pars peripheralis of orbicularis oris muscle
6 Tongue

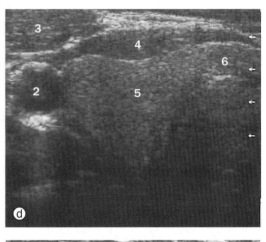

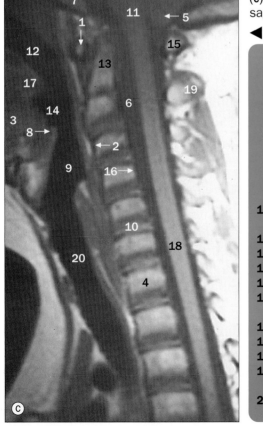

(c) Soft tissues of the neck, sagittal MR image. ◄

1 Anterior arch of atlas (first cervical vertebra)
2 Anterior longitudinal ligament
3 Base of tongue
4 Body of seventh cervical vertebra
5 Cerebellar tonsil
6 Cerebrospinal fluid
7 Clivus
8 Epiglottis
9 Hypopharynx
10 Intervertebral disc (between fifth and sixth cervical vertebrae)
11 Medulla oblongata
12 Nasopharynx
13 Odontoid process (dens)
14 Oropharynx
15 Posterior arch of atlas (first cervical vertebra)
16 Posterior longitudinal ligament
17 Soft palate
18 Spinal cord
19 Spinous process of axis (second cervical vertebra)
20 Trachea

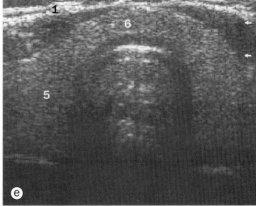

(d) and (e) Thyroid ultrasound, axial projection.

1 Deep cervical fascia
2 Internal jugular vein
3 Sternocleidomastoid muscle
4 Strap muscles of the neck
5 Thyroid gland
6 Thyroid isthmus

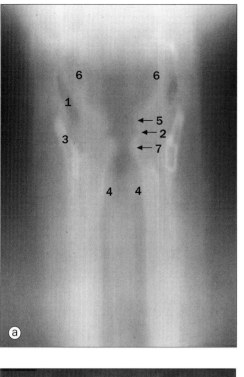

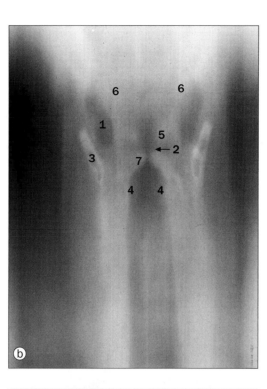

Tomography of the larynx, (a) at rest, (b) while phonating.

• Note how the vocal folds (7) move closer together during phonation.

1 Piriform fossa
2 Sinus of larynx
3 Thyroid cartilage
4 Trachea
5 Vestibular fold
6 Vestibule
7 Vocal fold

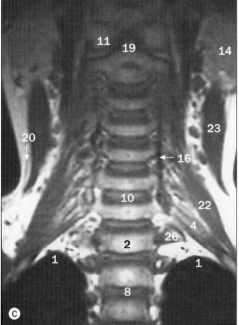

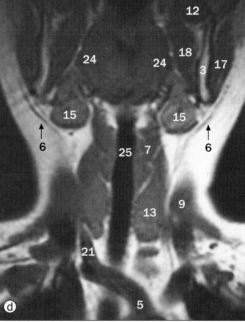

1 Apex of lung
2 Body of first thoracic vertebra
3 Body of mandible
4 Brachial plexus
5 Brachiocephalic trunk
6 Deep cervical fascia
7 Inferior constrictor muscle
8 Inferior end plate of second thoracic vertebra
9 Internal jugular vein
10 Intervertebral disc (between sixth and seventh cervical vertebrae)
11 Lateral mass of atlas (first cervical vertebra)
12 Lateral pterygoid muscle
13 Left lobe of thyroid gland
14 Left parotid gland
15 Left submandibular gland
16 Left vertebral artery
17 Masseter muscle
18 Medial pterygoid muscle
19 Odontoid process (dens)
20 Platysma muscle
21 Right common carotid artery
22 Scalenus medius muscle
23 Sternocleidomastoid muscle
24 Tongue
25 Trachea
26 Transverse process of first thoracic vertebra

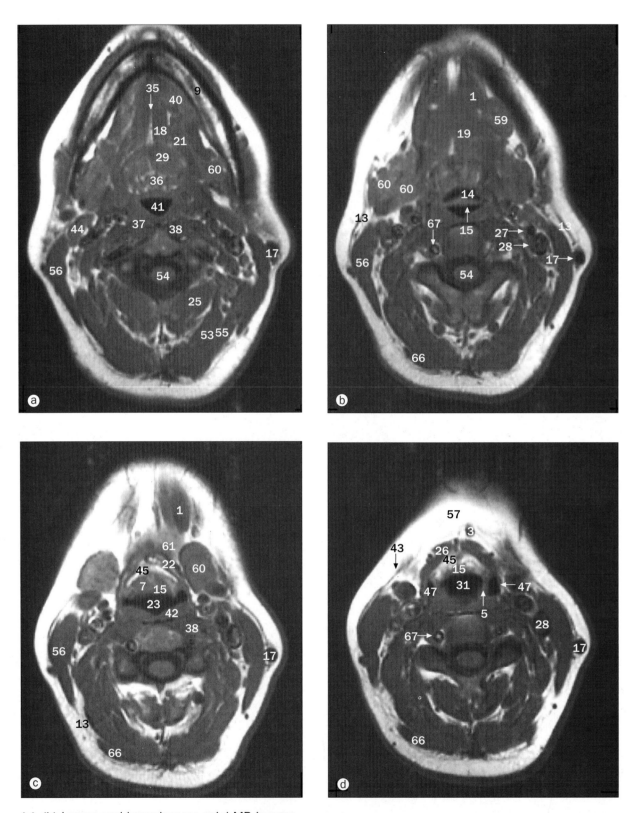

(a)–(h) Larynx and hypopharynx, axial MR images.

1 Anterior belly of digastric muscle	**9** Body of mandible	**17** External jugular vein
2 Anterior commissure	**10** Cervical oesophagus	**18** Genioglossus muscle
3 Anterior jugular vein	**11** Common carotid artery	**19** Geniohyoid muscle
4 Anterior margin of cricoid cartilage	**12** Cricothyroid joint	**20** Glottic space
5 Aryepiglottic fold	**13** Deep cervical fascia	**21** Hyoglossus muscle
6 Arytenoid cartilage	**14** Epiglottic valleculae	**22** Hyoid bone
7 Base of tongue and epiglottis	**15** Epiglottis	**23** Hypopharynx
8 Body of fifth cervical vertebra	**16** External carotid artery	**24** Inferior horn of thyroid cartilage

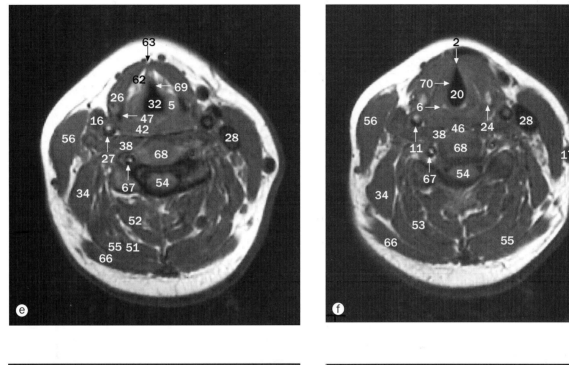

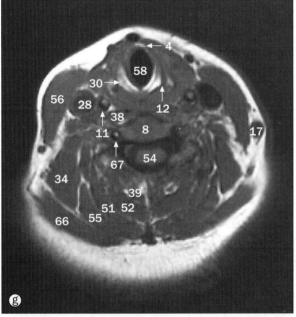

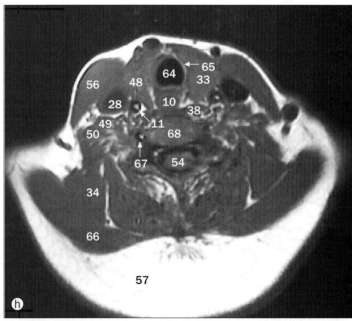

25 Inferior oblique muscle	41 Oropharynx	56 Sternocleidomastoid muscle
26 Infrahyoid muscle	42 Pharyngeal constrictor	57 Subcutaneous fat
27 Internal carotid artery	43 Platysma muscle	58 Subglottic space
28 Internal jugular vein	44 Posterior belly of digastric muscle	59 Sublingual gland
29 Intrinsic tongue muscle	45 Pre-epiglottic space	60 Submandibular gland
30 Lamina of cricoid cartilage	46 Prevertebral space	61 Suprahyoid muscles
31 Laryngeal inlet	47 Pyriform sinus	62 Thyroid cartilage
32 Laryngeal vestibule	48 Right lobe of thyroid	63 Thyroid notch
33 Left lobe of thyroid	49 Scalenus anterior muscle	64 Trachea
34 Levator scapulae muscle	50 Scalenus medius and posterior muscles	65 Tracheal ring
35 Lingual septum		66 Trapezius muscle
36 Lingual tonsils	51 Semispinalis capitis muscle	67 Vertebral artery
37 Longus capitis muscle	52 Semispinalis cervicis muscle	68 Vertebral body
38 Longus colli muscle	53 Semispinalis muscle	69 Vestibular fold (false cord)
39 Multifidus muscle	54 Spinal cord	70 Vocal cord
40 Mylohyoid muscle	55 Splenius capitis muscle	

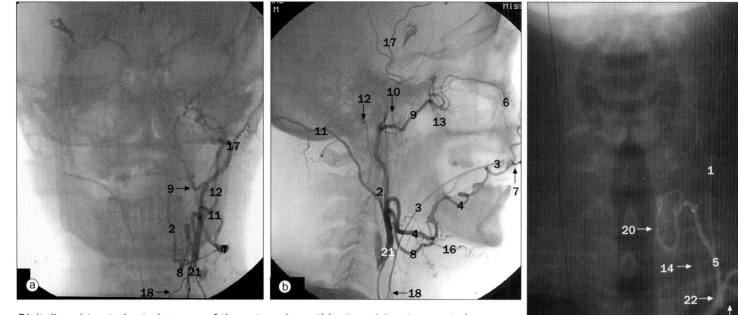

Digitally subtracted arteriograms of the external carotid artery, (a) anteroposterior projection, (b) lateral projection. (c) Thyroid arteriogram.

1 Ascending cervical artery	11 Occipital artery	19 Suprascapular artery
2 Ascending pharyngeal artery	12 Posterior auricular artery	20 Thyroid branches of
3 Endotracheal tube	13 Posterior superior alveolar	inferior thyroid artery
4 Facial artery	artery	21 Tip of catheter in
5 Inferior thyroid artery	14 Reflux of contrast into	externalcarotid artery
6 Infra-orbital artery	vertebral artery	22 Tip of catheter in
7 Labial branch of facial artery	15 Subclavian artery	thyrocervical trunk
8 Lingual artery	16 Submental artery	23 Transverse cervical artery
9 Maxillary artery	17 Superficial temporal artery	
10 Middle meningeal artery	18 Superior thyroid artery	

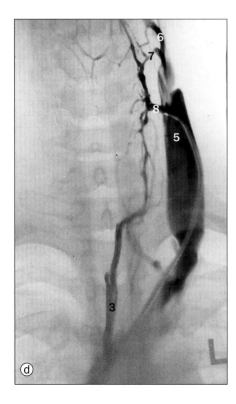

(d) Neck venogram, (e) MR angiogram of neck vessels.

1 Common carotid artery
2 External carotid artery
3 Inferior thyroid vein
4 Internal carotid artery
5 Internal jugular vein
6 Lingual vein
7 Superior thyroid vein
8 Tip of catheter in middle thyroid vein
9 Vertebral artery

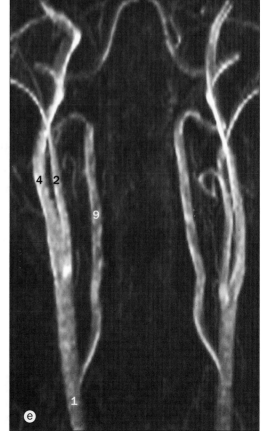

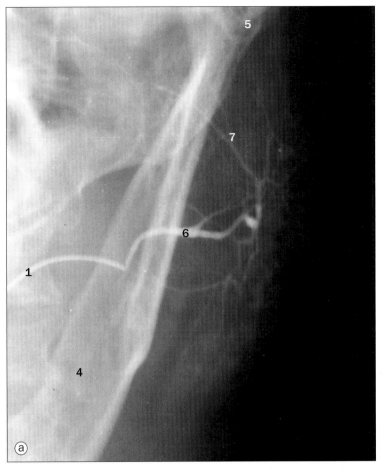

(a) Parotid sialogram.   ▲

1 Catheter	**4** Mandible
2 Coronoid process of	**5** Mastoid process
mandible	**6** Parotid (Stensen's) duct
3 Hyoid bone	**7** Secondary ductules

(c) Parotid sialogram, submentovertical projection. ▼

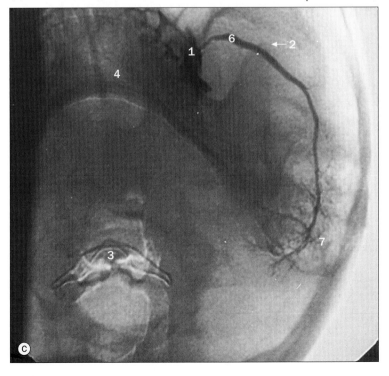

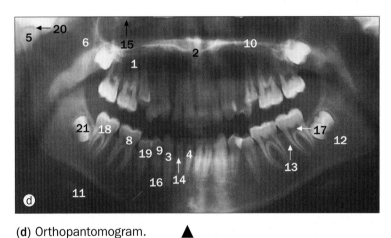

(b) Submandibular sialogram.   ▲

1 Catheter
2 Main submandibular (Wharton's) duct
3 Mandible
4 Secondary ductules

(d) Orthopantomogram.   ▲

1 Alveolar process of maxilla	**12** Inferior alveolar canal
2 Anterior nasal spine	**13** Lamina propria
3 Canine	**14** Lateral incisor
4 Central incisor	**15** Maxillary sinus (antrum)
5 Condyle of mandible	**16** Mental foramen
6 Coronoid process of mandible	**17** Pulp chamber
7 External acoustic meatus	**18** Second molar
8 First molar	**19** Second premolar
9 First premolar	**20** Temporomandibular joint
10 Hard palate	**21** Third molar
11 Hyoid bone	

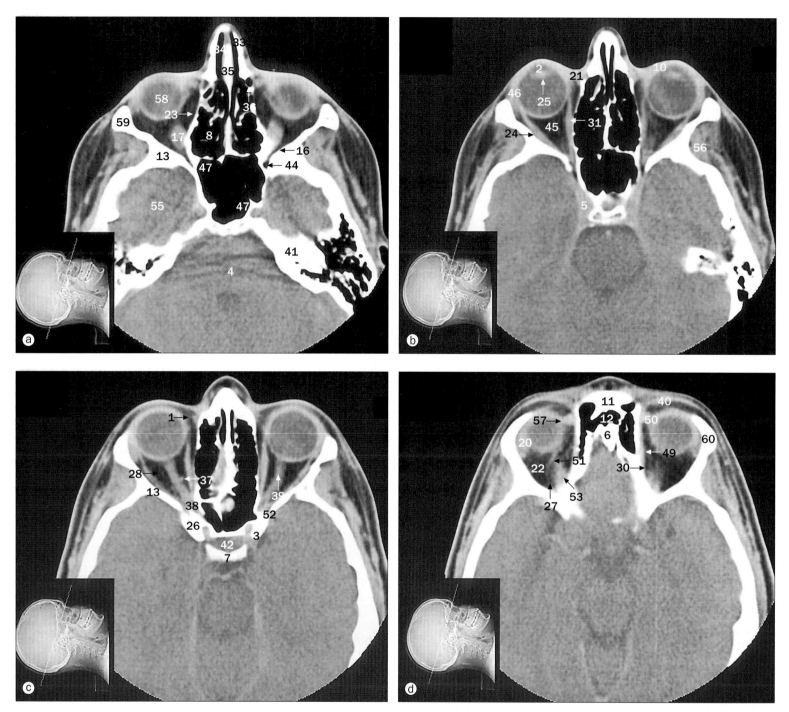

Orbits, axial CT images are demonstrated at the following levels: (a) inferior orbit and globe; (b) mid orbit below the optic nerve; (c) mid orbit at the level of the optic nerve; (d) superior orbit.

1	Angular vein	**11**	Frontal bone	**21**	Lacrimal sac
2	Anterior chamber	**12**	Frontal sinus	**22**	Lacrimal vein
3	Anterior clinoid process	**13**	Greater wing of sphenoid	**23**	Lamina papyracea
4	Brainstem	**14**	Inferior nasal concha (turbinate)	**24**	Lateral rectus muscle
5	Cavernous sinus	**15**	Inferior oblique muscle	**25**	Lens
6	Crista galli	**16**	Inferior orbital fissure	**26**	Lesser wing of sphenoid
7	Dorsum sellae	**17**	Inferior rectus muscle	**27**	Levator palpebrae superioris muscle
8	Ethmoidal sinuses	**18**	Infra-orbital canal	**28**	Long posterior ciliary artery
9	Ethmoidal sinuses (posterior)	**19**	Infra-orbital margin	**29**	Maxillary sinus (antrum)
10	Eyelid	**20**	Lacrimal gland	**30**	Medial ophthalmic vein

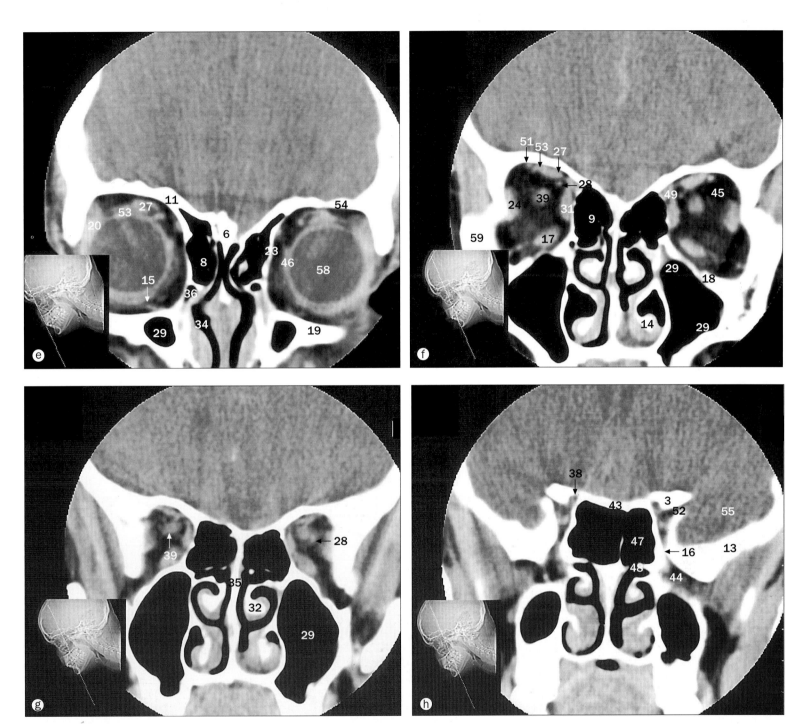

Orbits, coronal CT images are demonstrated at the following levels: (e) globe, (f) mid orbit, (g) posterior orbit, (h) superior and inferior orbital fissures.

31 Medial rectus muscle	**41** Petrous ridge	**51** Superior ophthalmic vein
32 Middle nasal concha (turbinate)	**42** Pituitary gland	**52** Superior orbital fissure
33 Nasal bone	**43** Planum sphenoidale	**53** Superior rectus muscle
34 Nasal cavity	**44** Pterygopalatine fossa	**54** Supra-orbital margin
35 Nasal septum	**45** Retrobulbar fat	**55** Temporal lobe
36 Nasolacrimal duct	**46** Sclera	**56** Temporalis muscle
37 Ophthalmic artery	**47** Sphenoidal sinus	**57** Trochlea of superior oblique muscle
38 Optic canal	**48** Superior nasal concha (turbinate)	**58** Vitreous
39 Optic nerve	**49** Superior oblique muscle	**59** Zygomatic bone
40 Orbicularis muscle	**50** Superior oblique tendon	**60** Zygomatic process of frontal bone

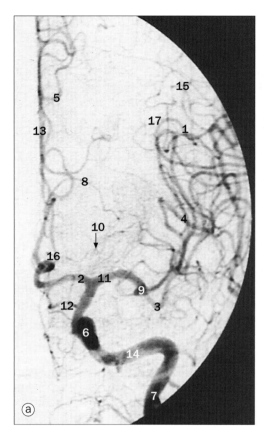

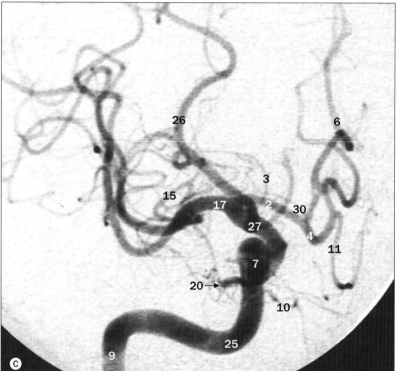

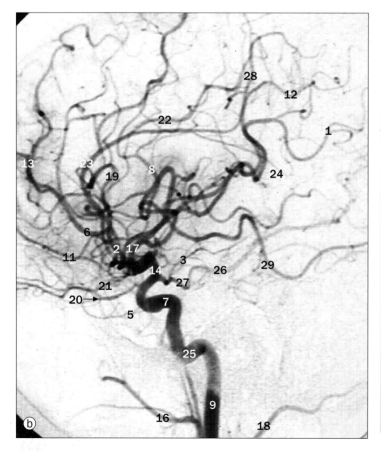

1 Angular branches of middle cerebral artery
2 Anterior cerebral artery
3 Anterior temporal branches of middle cerebral artery
4 Branches (in insula) of middle cerebral artery
5 Callosomarginal artery
6 Cavernous portion of internal carotid artery
7 Cervical portion of internal carotid artery
8 Frontopolar artery
9 Genu of middle cerebral artery
10 Lenticulostriate arteries
11 Middle cerebral artery
12 Orbitofrontal branch of pericallosal artery
13 Pericallosal artery
14 Petrous portion of internal carotid artery
15 Posterior parietal branches of middle cerebral artery
16 Recurrent artery of Heubner
17 Sylvian point

Digitally subtracted arterial phase of carotid arteriograms,
(a) anteroposterior projection, (b) lateral projection, (c) oblique
projection.

1 Angular artery
2 Anterior cerebral artery
3 Anterior choroidal artery
4 Anterior communicating artery
5 Anterior temporal artery
6 Callosomarginal artery
7 Cavernous portion of internal carotid artery
8 Central sulcus artery
9 Cervical portion of internal carotid artery
10 Ethmoidal branch of ophthalmic artery
11 Frontopolar artery
12 Inferior internal parietal artery
13 Internal frontal branch of anterior cerebral artery
14 Intracranial (supraclinoid) internal carotid artery
15 Lenticulostriate artery
16 Maxillary artery
17 Middle cerebral artery
18 Occipital artery
19 Operculofrontal artery
20 Ophthalmic artery
21 Orbitofrontal artery
22 Paracentral artery
23 Pericallosal artery
24 Pericallosal artery extending around corpus callosum
25 Petrous portion of internal carotid artery
26 Posterior cerebral artery
27 Posterior communicating artery
28 Posterior parietal artery
29 Posterior temporal artery
30 Recurrent artery of Heubner

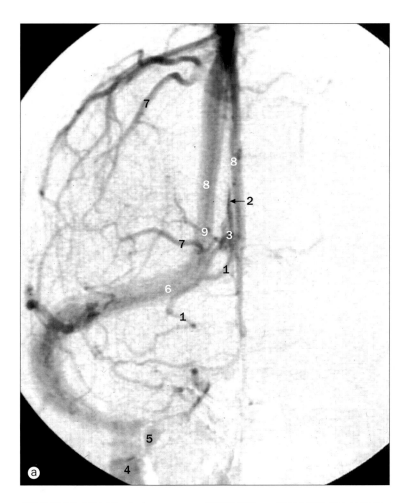

(a) Digitally subtracted venous phase of carotid arteriogram, anteroposterior projection.

1	Basal vein of Rosenthal
2	Inferior sagittal sinus
3	Internal cerebral vein
4	Internal jugular vein
5	Jugular bulb
6	Right transverse sinus
7	Superficial cortical veins
8	Superior sagittal sinus
9	Thalamostriate vein

(b) Digitally subtracted venous phase of carotid arteriogram, lateral projection.

1	Anterior caudate vein
2	Basal vein of Rosenthal
3	Cavernous sinus
4	Confluence of venous sinuses (torcular Herophili)
5	Great cerebral vein of Galen
6	Inferior sagittal sinus
7	Internal cerebral vein
8	Internal jugular vein
9	Sigmoid sinus
10	Sphenoparietal sinus
11	Straight sinus
12	Superficial cerebral veins
13	Superior sagittal sinus
14	Thalamostriate vein
15	Transverse sinus
16	Vein of Labbé
17	Vein of Trolard
18	Venous angle

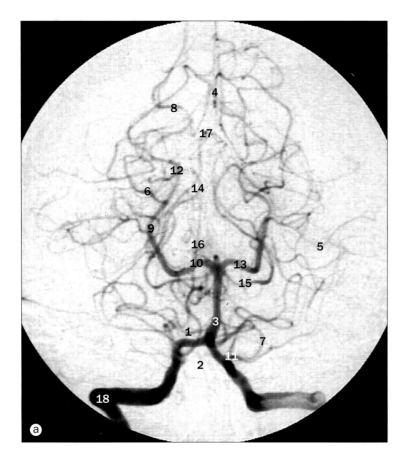

(a) Digitally subtracted arterial phase of vertebral arteriogram, anteroposterior projection.

 1 Anterior inferior cerebellar artery
 2 Anterior spinal artery
 3 Basilar artery
 4 Calcarine artery
 5 Hemispheric branch of superior cerebellar artery
 6 Inferior temporal artery
 7 Medullary segment of posterior inferior cerebellar artery
 8 Parieto-occipital artery
 9 Posterior cerebral artery in ambient cistern
10 Posterior cerebral artery in interpeduncular cistern
11 Posterior inferior cerebellar artery
12 Quadrigeminal portion of posterior cerebral artery
13 Site of junction with posterior communicating artery
14 Superior cerebellar arteries behind brainstem
15 Superior cerebellar artery
16 Thalamoperforating branches of superior cerebellar artery
17 Vermian branch of superior cerebellar artery
18 Vertebral artery exiting transverse foramen of atlas
     (first cervical vertebra)

(b) Digitally subtracted arterial phase of vertebral arteriogram, lateral projection.

 1 Anterior inferior cerebellar artery
 2 Anterior medullary segment of posterior inferior cerebellar artery
 3 Basilar artery
 4 Calcarine artery
 5 Hemispheric branches of posterior inferior cerebellar artery
 6 Inferior vermian segment of posterior inferior cerebellar artery
 7 Lateral medullary segment of posterior inferior cerebellar artery
 8 Meningeal branch of vertebral artery
 9 Origin of posterior inferior cerebellar artery
10 Parieto-occipital artery
11 Posterior cerebral artery
12 Posterior choroidal branches of posterior cerebral artery
13 Posterior medullary segment of posterior inferior cerebellar artery
14 Posterior temporal artery
15 Retrotonsillar segment of posterior inferior cerebellar artery
16 Splenial branches of posterior cerebral artery
17 Superior cerebellar artery
18 Supratonsillar segment of posterior inferior cerebellar artery
19 Thalamoperforate branches of posterior cerebral artery
20 Vertebral artery
21 Vertebral artery exiting transverse foramen of atlas
     (first cervical vertebra)

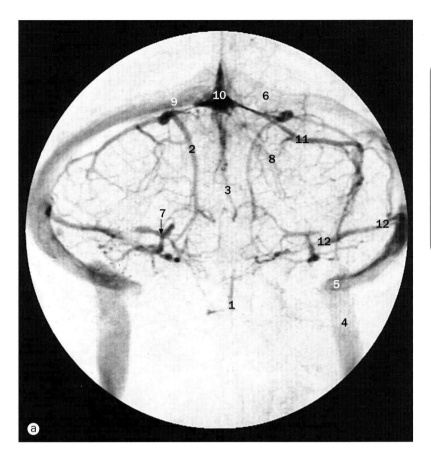

(a) Digitally subtracted venous phase of vertebral arteriogram, anteroposterior projection.

1 Anterior pontomesencephalic vein
2 Inferior hemispheric vein
3 Inferior vermian vein
4 Internal jugular vein
5 Jugular bulb
6 Left transverse sinus
7 Petrosal vein
8 Posterior mesencephalic vein
9 Right transverse sinus
10 Straight sinus
11 Superior hemispheric vein
12 Superior petrosal sinus

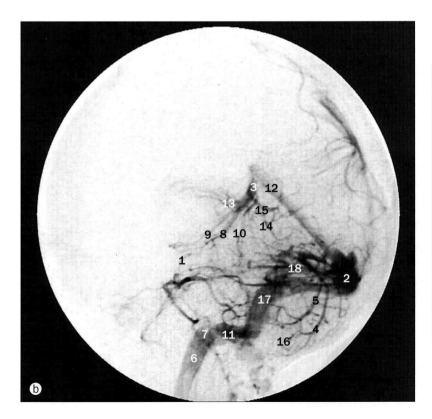

(b) Digitally subtracted venous phase of vertebral arteriogram, lateral projection.

1 Anterior pontomesencephalic vein
2 Confluence of venous sinuses (torcular Herophili)
3 Great cerebral vein of Galen
4 Inferior hemispheric vein
5 Inferior vermian vein
6 Internal jugular vein
7 Jugular bulb
8 Lateral mesencephalic vein
9 Posterior mesencephalic vein
10 Precentral cerebellar vein
11 Sigmoid sinus
12 Straight sinus
13 Superior choroidal vein
14 Superior hemispheric vein
15 Superior vermian vein
16 Tonsillar vein
17 Transverse sinus
18 Vein of the great horizontal fissure

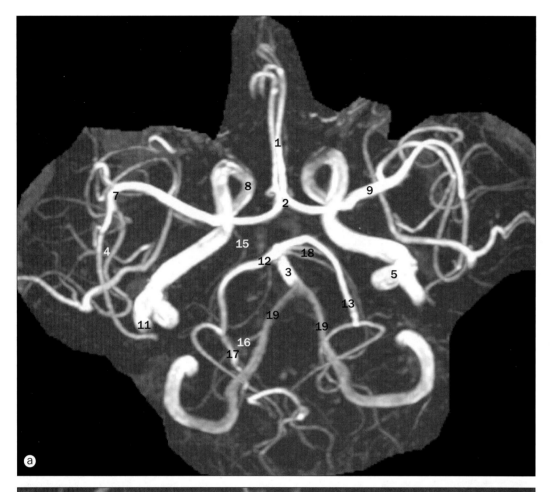

1 Anterior cerebral artery
2 Anterior communicating artery
3 Basilar artery
4 Branches (in insula) of middle cerebral artery
5 Cavernous portion of internal carotid artery
6 Cervical portion of internal carotid artery
7 Genu of middle cerebral artery
8 Intracranial (supraclinoid) internal carotid artery
9 Middle cerebral artery
10 Ophthalmic artery
11 Petrous portion of internal carotid artery
12 Posterior cerebral artery
13 Posterior cerebral artery in ambient cistern
14 Posterior cerebral artery in interpeduncular cistern
15 Posterior communicating artery
16 Posterior inferior cerebellar artery
17 Quadrigeminal portion of posterior cerebral artery
18 Superior cerebellar artery
19 Vertebral artery

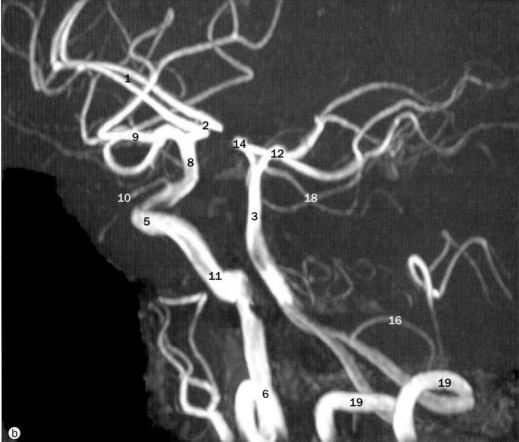

Circle of Willis, arteries of the brain with MRA, **(a)** axial and **(b)** lateral projection.

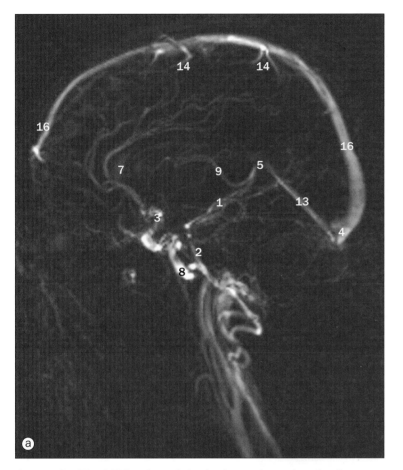

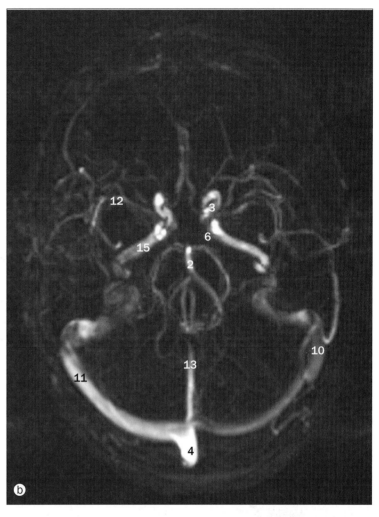

Circle of Willis, MRA veins of the brain, (a) lateral projection, (b) axial projection.

1 Basal vein of Rosenthal	**9** Internal cerebral vein
2 Basilar artery	**10** Left transverse sinus
3 Cavernous sinus	**11** Right transverse sinus
4 Confluence of venous sinuses (torcular Herophili)	**12** Sphenoparietal sinus
5 Great cerebral vein of Galen	**13** Straight sinus
6 Inferior petrosal sinus	**14** Superficial cerebral veins
7 Inferior sagittal sinus	**15** Superior petrosal sinus
8 Internal carotid artery	**16** Superior sagittal sinus

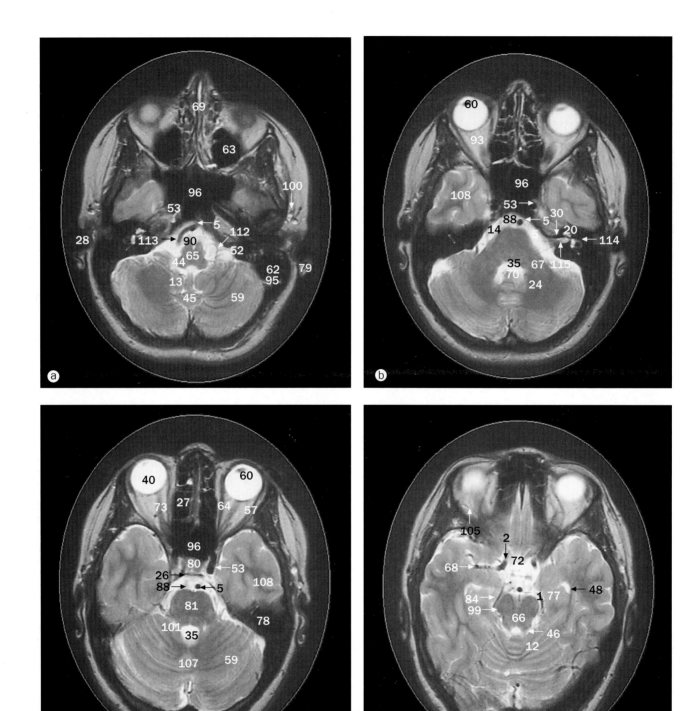

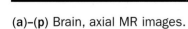
(a)–(p) Brain, axial MR images.

1 Ambient cistern	**11** Centrum semi ovale	**21** Confluence of venous sinuses
2 Anterior cerebral artery	**12** Cerebellar folia	(torcular Herophili)
3 Anterior limb of internal capsule	**13** Cerebellar tonsil	**22** Corona radiata
4 Aqueduct of Sylvius	**14** Cerebellopontine cistern	**23** Cortical vein
5 Basilar artery	**15** Cerebral peduncle	**24** Dentate nucleus
6 Body of lateral ventricle	**16** Choroid plexus in trigone of	**25** Diploë
7 Branch of middle cerebral artery	lateral ventricle	**26** Dorsum sellae
in lateral sulcus (Sylvian fissure)	**17** Choroid vessels	**27** Ethmoidal air cells
8 Callosomarginal artery	**18** Cingulate gyrus	**28** External acoustic meatus
9 Caudate nucleus	**19** Claustrum	**29** External capsule
10 Central sulcus of Rolando	**20** Cochlea	**30** Facial nerve in internal acoustic canal

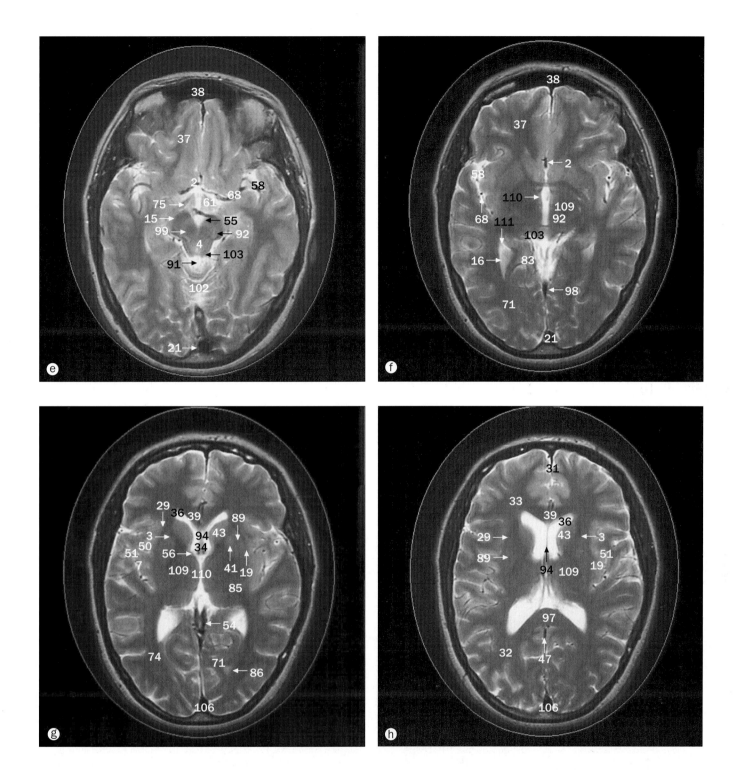

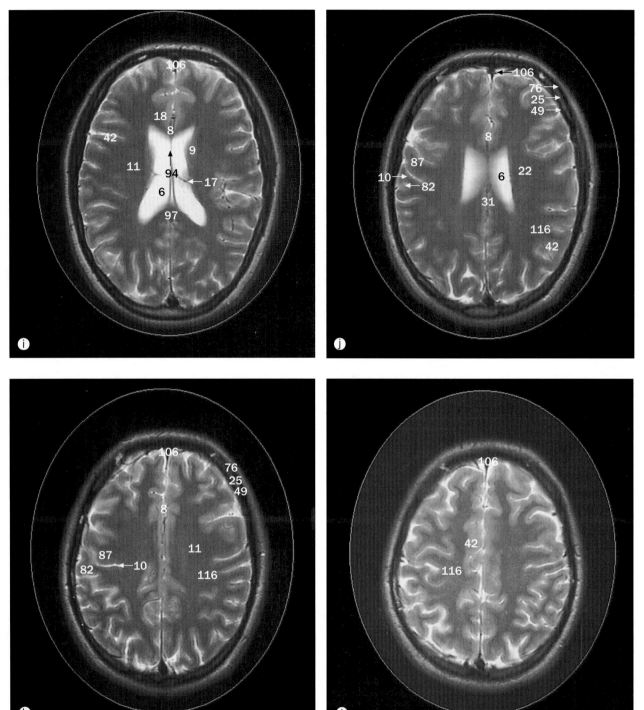

(i)–(p) Brain, axial MR images.

61	Mammillary bodies in suprasellar cistern	**73**	Optic nerve	**85**	Posterior limb of internal capsule
62	Mastoid air cells	**74**	Optic radiations	**86**	Posterior (occipital) horn of lateral ventricle
63	Maxillary sinus (antrum)	**75**	Optic tract		
64	Medial rectus muscle	**76**	Outer table	**87**	Precentral gyrus
65	Medulla oblongata	**77**	Parahippocampal gyrus	**88**	Prepontine cistern
66	Mesencephalon (midbrain)	**78**	Petrous temporal bone	**89**	Putamen
67	Middle cerebellar peduncle	**79**	Pinna of ear	**90**	Pyramid of medulla oblongata
68	Middle cerebral artery	**80**	Pituitary gland	**91**	Quadrigeminal cistern
69	Nasal septum	**81**	Pons	**92**	Red nucleus
70	Nodule of cerebellum	**82**	Postcentral gyrus	**93**	Retro-orbital fat
71	Occipital lobe	**83**	Posterior cerebral artery	**94**	Septum pellucidum
72	Optic chiasma in suprasellar cistern	**84**	Posterior cerebral artery in ambient cistern	**95**	Sigmoid sinus

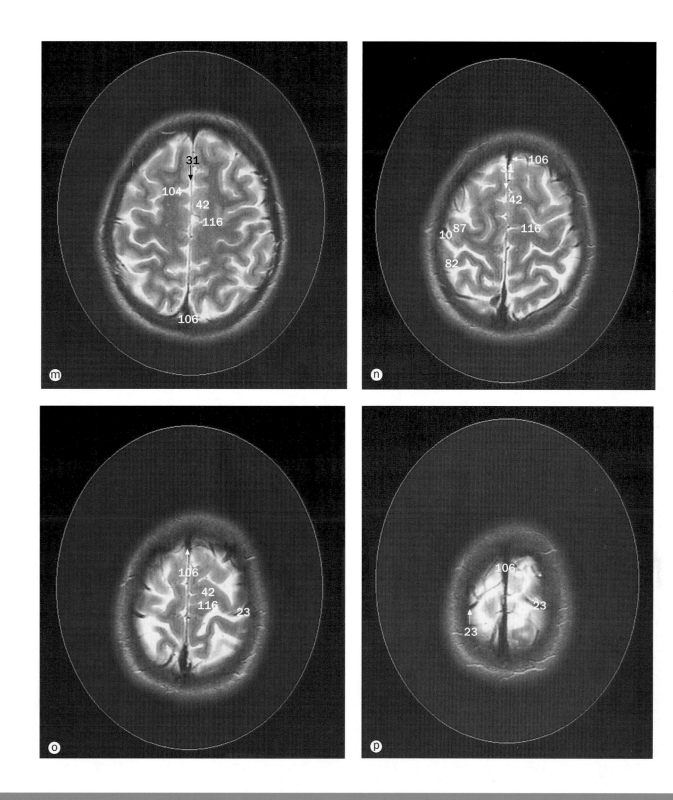

96 Sphenoidal sinus
97 Splenium of corpus callosum
98 Straight sinus
99 Substantia nigra
100 Superficial temporal artery
101 Superior cerebellar peduncle
102 Superior cerebellar vermis
103 Superior colliculus
104 Superior frontal gyrus
105 Superior ophthalmic vein
106 Superior sagittal sinus

107 Superior vermis
108 Temporal lobe
109 Thalamus
110 Third ventricle
111 Trigone of lateral ventricle
112 Vagus nerve
113 Vertebral artery
114 Vestibular part of inner ear
115 Vestibulocochlear nerve in internal acoustic canal
116 White matter

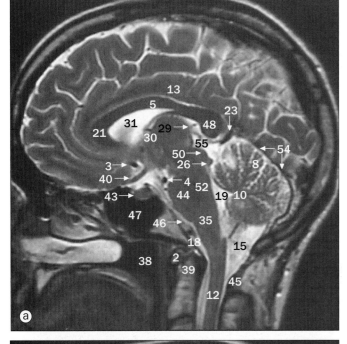

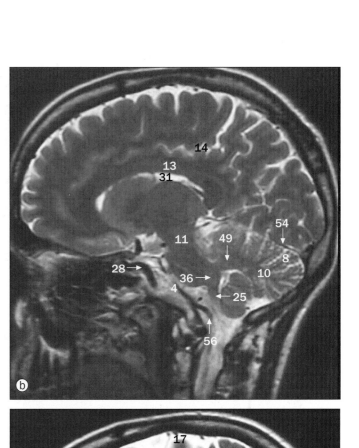

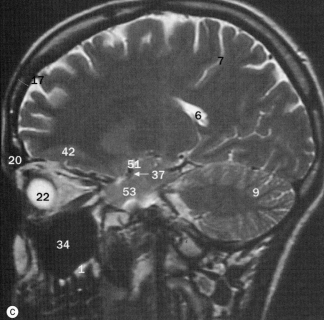

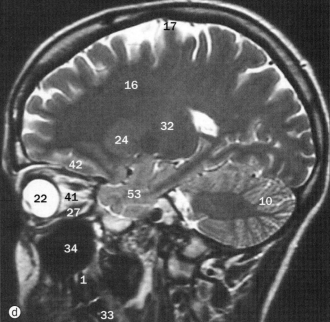

(a)–(d) Brain, sagittal MR images.

1 Alveolar ridge	15 Cisterna magna	29 Internal cerebral vein	43 Pituitary gland
2 Anterior arch of atlas	(cerebellomedullary cistern)	30 Interventricular foramen	44 Pons
(first cervical vertebra)	16 Corona radiata	of Monro	45 Posterior arch of atlas
3 Anterior cerebral artery	17 Cortical vein	31 Lateral ventricle	46 Prepontine cistern
4 Basilar artery	18 Foramen magnum	32 Lentiform nucleus	47 Sphenoidal sinus
5 Body of corpus callosum	19 Fourth ventricle	33 Mandible	48 Splenium of corpus callosum
6 Body of lateral ventricle	20 Frontal sinus	34 Maxillary sinus (antrum)	49 Superior cerebellar peduncle
7 Central sulcus of Rolando	21 Genu of corpus callosum	35 Medulla oblongata	50 Superior colliculus
8 Cerebellar folia	22 Globe	36 Middle cerebellar peduncle	51 Sylvian fissure
9 Cerebellar hemisphere	23 Great cerebral vein of Galen	37 Middle cerebral artery	52 Tegmentum of pons
10 Cerebellum	24 Head of caudate nucleus	38 Nasopharynx	53 Temporal lobe of brain
11 Cerebral peduncle	25 Inferior cerebellar peduncle	39 Odontoid process (dens)	54 Tentorium cerebelli
12 Cervical spinal cord	26 Inferior colliculus	40 Optic chiasma in	55 Third ventricle
13 Cingulate gyrus	27 Inferior rectus muscle	suprasellarcistern	56 Vertebral artery
14 Cingulate sulcus	28 Internal carotid artery in	41 Optic nerve	
	cavernous sinus	42 Orbital cortex of frontal lobe	

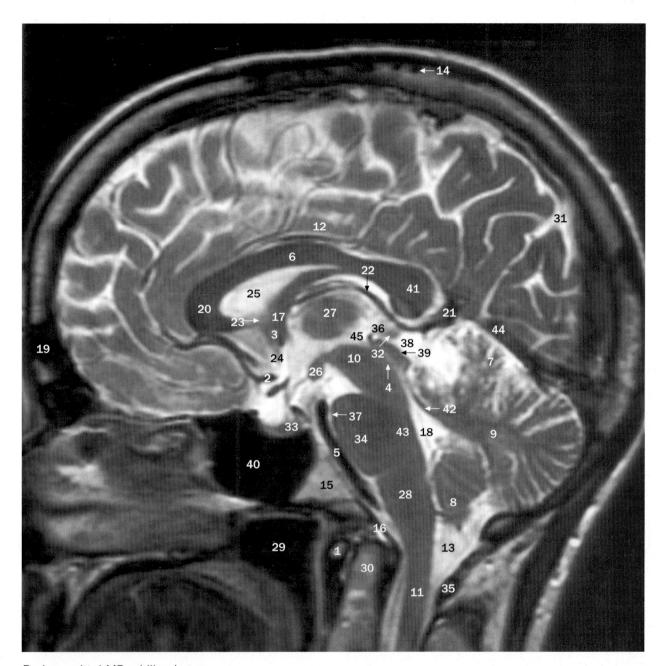

Brain, sagittal MR midline image.

1 Anterior arch of atlas (first cervical vertebra)	**15** Fat in marrow of clivus	**31** Parieto-occipital fissure
2 Anterior cerebral artery	**16** Foramen magnum	**32** Pineal gland
3 Anterior commissure	**17** Fornix	**33** Pituitary gland
4 Aqueduct of Sylvius	**18** Fourth ventricle	**34** Pons
5 Basilar artery	**19** Frontal sinus	**35** Posterior arch of atlas
6 Body of corpus callosum	**20** Genu of corpus callosum	**36** Posterior commissure
7 Cerebellar folia	**21** Great cerebral vein of Galen	**37** Prepontine cistern
8 Cerebellar tonsil	**22** Internal cerebral vein	**38** Quadrigeminal cistern
9 Cerebellum	**23** Interventricular foramen of Monro	**39** Quadrigeminal plate of midbrain
10 Cerebral peduncles of midbrain	**24** Lamina terminalis	**40** Sphenoidal sinus
11 Cervical spinal cord	**25** Lateral ventricle	**41** Splenium of corpus callosum
12 Cingulate gyrus	**26** Mammillary body	**42** Superior medullary velum
13 Cisterna magna (cerebellomedullary cistern)	**27** Massa intermedia	**43** Tegmentum of pons
	28 Medulla oblongata	**44** Tentorium cerebelli
14 Diploic veins	**29** Nasopharynx	**45** Third ventricle
	30 Odontoid process (dens)	

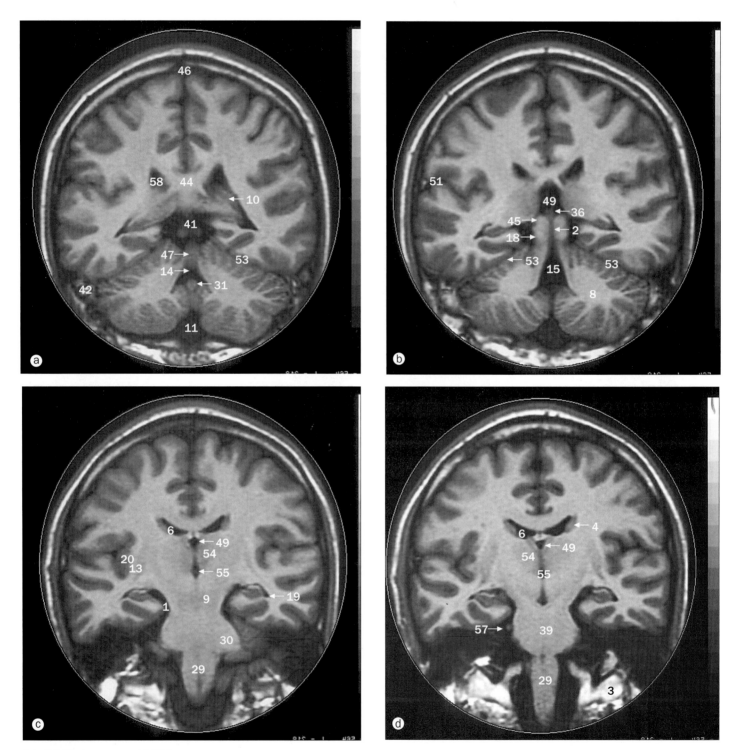

(a)–(h) Brain, coronal MR images.

1 Ambient cistern	**11** Cisterna magna (cerebellomedullary cistern)	**21** Interhemispheric cistern
2 Aqueduct of Sylvius	**12** Claustrum and external capsule	**22** Internal capsule
3 Atlas (first cervical vertebra)	**13** External capsule	**23** Interpeduncular cistern
4 Body of caudate nucleus	**14** Fornix	**24** Intracavernous internal carotid artery
5 Body of corpus callosum	**15** Fourth ventricle	**25** Lateral ventricle
6 Body of lateral ventricle	**16** Head of caudate nucleus	**26** Lentiform nucleus
7 Cavum septum pellucidum	**17** Hippocampus	**27** Mandible
8 Cerebellar hemisphere	**18** Inferior colliculus	**28** Marrow of basisphenoid (clivus)
9 Cerebral peduncle	**19** Inferior (temporal) horn of lateral ventricle	**29** Medulla oblongata
10 Choroid plexus	**20** Insula	**30** Middle cerebellar peduncle

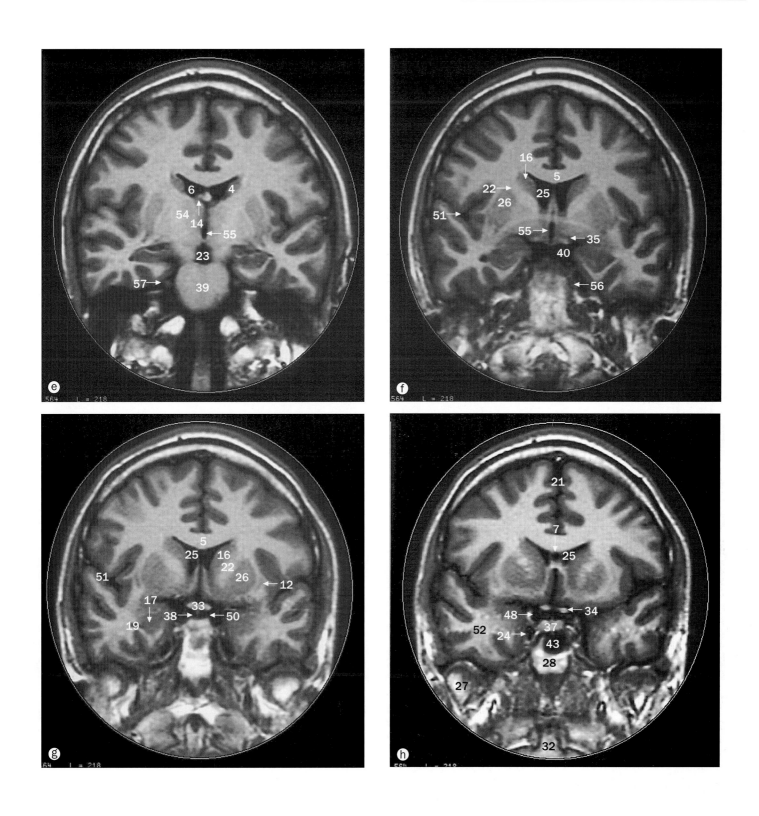

31 Nodule of cerebellum	**41** Quadrigeminal cistern	**51** Sylvian fissure
32 Odontoid process (dens)	**42** Sigmoid sinus	**52** Temporal lobe
33 Optic chiasma in suprasellar cistern	**43** Sphenoidal sinus	**53** Tentorium cerebelli
34 Optic nerve	**44** Splenium of corpus callosum	**54** Thalamus
35 Optic tract	**45** Superior colliculus	**55** Third ventricle
36 Pineal gland	**46** Superior sagittal sinus	**56** Trigeminal (gasserian) ganglion in recess
37 Pituitary gland	**47** Superior vermis	(Meckel's cave)
38 Pituitary stalk in suprasellar cistern	**48** Supraclinoid internal carotid artery	**57** Trigeminal nerve
39 Pons	**49** Suprapineal recess of the third ventricle	**58** Trigone of lateral ventricle
40 Prepontine cistern	**50** Suprasellar cistern	

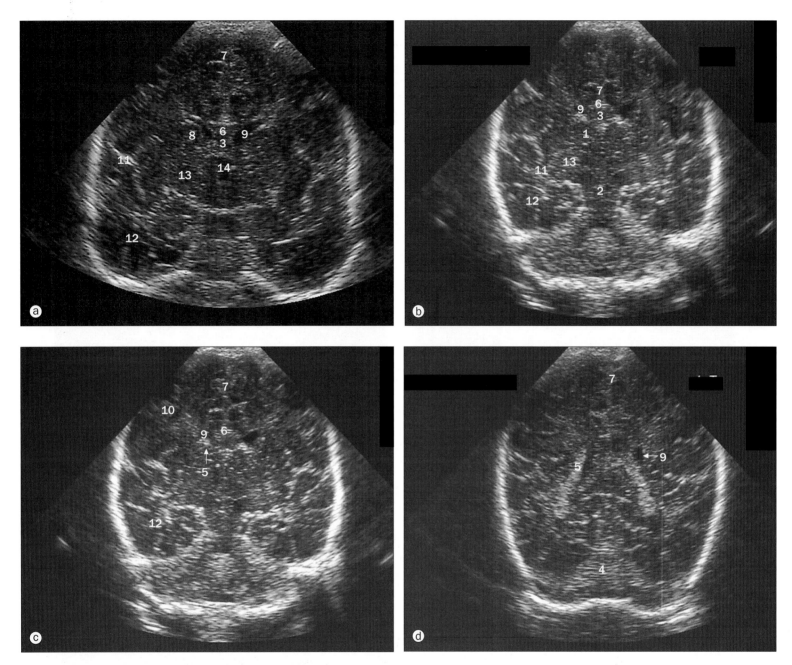

(a)–(d) Neonatal brain, coronal ultrasound images.

1 Body of caudate nucleus
2 Brainstem
3 Cavum septum pellucidum
4 Cerebellum
5 Choroid plexus
6 Corpus callosum
7 Falx cerebri
8 Head of caudate nucleus
9 Lateral ventricle
10 Parietal lobe of brain
11 Sylvian fissure
12 Temporal lobe
13 Thalamus
14 Third ventricle

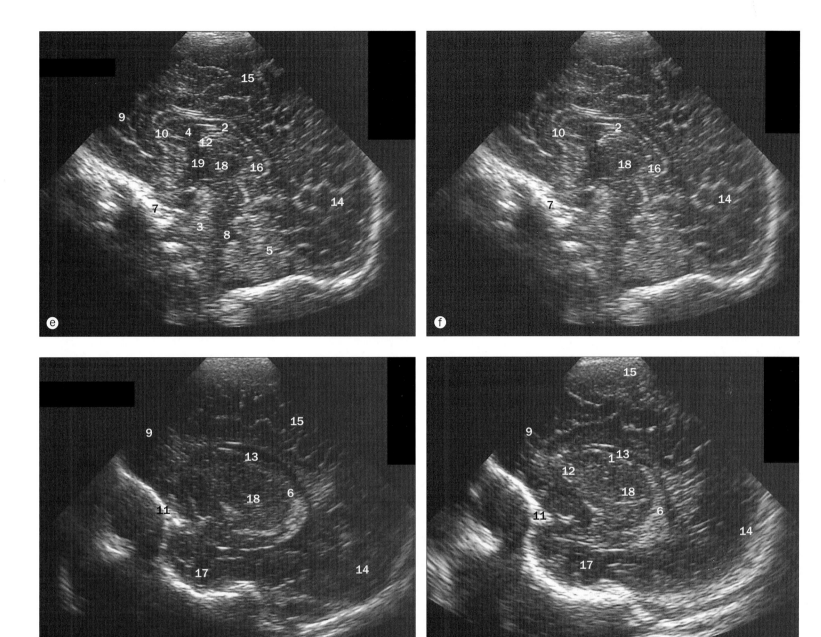

(e)–(h) Neonatal brain, sagittal ultrasound images.

1 Body of caudate nucleus	11 Greater wing of sphenoid
2 Body of corpus callosum	12 Head of caudate nucleus
3 Brainstem	13 Lateral ventricle
4 Cavum septum pellucidum	14 Occipital lobe
5 Cerebellum	15 Parietal lobe of brain
6 Choroid plexus	16 Splenium of corpus callosum
7 Clivus	17 Temporal lobe
8 Fourth ventricle	18 Thalamus
9 Frontal lobe	19 Third ventricle
10 Genu of corpus callosum	

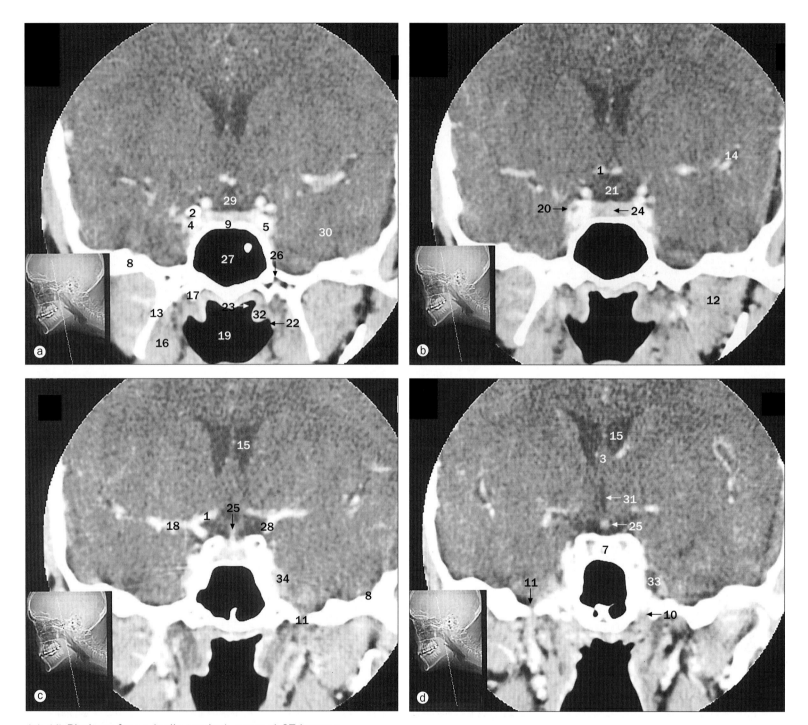

(a)–(d) Pituitary fossa (sella turcica), coronal CT images.
These images show 2 mm coronal slices through the sella turcica (pituitary fossa) from anterior **(a)** to posterior **(d)** during the intravenous infusion of non-ionic water-soluble contrast medium.

1 Anterior cerebral artery	**13** Lateral pterygoid plate	**24** Pituitary gland
2 Anterior clinoid process	**14** Lateral sulcus (Sylvian fissure) with	**25** Pituitary stalk
3 Body of fornix	branches of middle cerebral artery	**26** Pterygoid (vidian) canal
4 Cavernous carotid artery	**15** Lateral ventricle	**27** Sphenoidal sinus
5 Cavernous sinus	**16** Medial pterygoid muscle	**28** Supraclinoid internal carotid artery
6 Choroid plexus	**17** Medial pterygoid plate	**29** Suprasellar cistern
7 Dorsum sellae	**18** Middle cerebral artery	**30** Temporal lobe of brain
8 Floor of middle cranial fossa	**19** Nasopharynx	**31** Third ventricle
9 Floor of pituitary fossa (sella turcica)	**20** Oculomotor nerve	**32** Torus tubarius
10 Foramen lacerum	**21** Optic chiasma	**33** Trigeminal (gasserian) ganglion in recess
11 Foramen ovale	**22** Orifice of auditory (Eustachian) tube	(Meckel's cave)
12 Lateral pterygoid muscle	**23** Pharyngeal recess (fossa of Rosenmuller)	**34** Trigeminal nerve

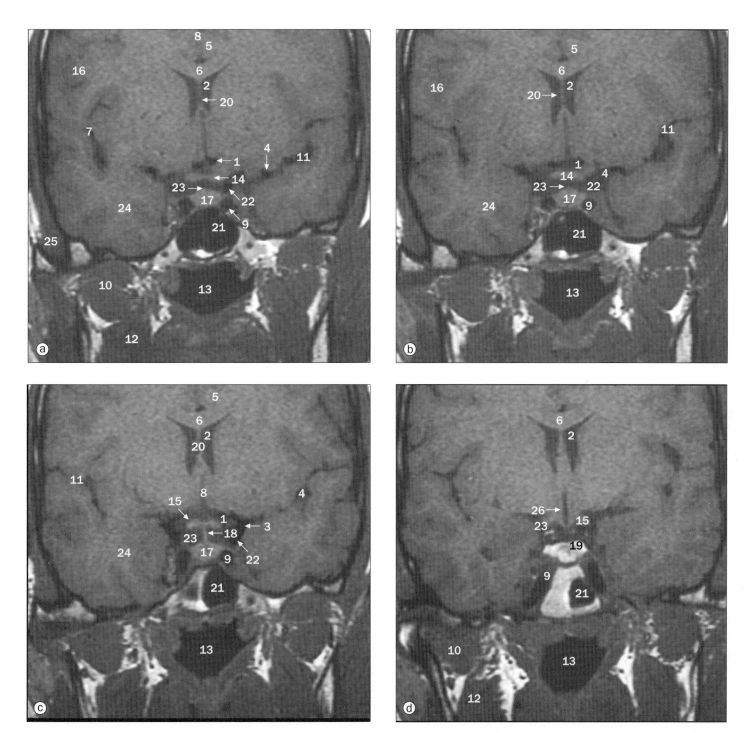

Pituitary fossa (sella turcica), coronal MR images), (a) at the level of the anterior clinoid, (b) mid fossa, (c) at the level of the pituitary stalk, (d) at the level of the dorsum sellae.

1	Anterior cerebral artery	9	Internal carotid artery in cavernous sinus
2	Anterior horn of lateral ventricle	10	Lateral pterygoid muscle
3	Bifurcation of internal carotid artery	11	Lateral sulcus (Sylvian fissure)
4	Branch of middle cerebral artery in lateral sulcus (Sylvian fissure)	12	Medial pterygoid muscle
5	Cingulate gyrus	13	Nasopharynx
6	Corpus callosum	14	Optic chiasma
7	Insula	15	Optic tract
8	Interhemispheric fissure	16	Parietal lobe of brain
		17	Pituitary gland
18	Pituitary stalk		
19	Posterior clinoid process		
20	Septum pellucidum		
21	Sphenoidal sinus		
22	Supraclinoid carotid artery		
23	Suprasellar cistern		
24	Temporal lobe of brain		
25	Temporalis muscle		
26	Third ventricle		

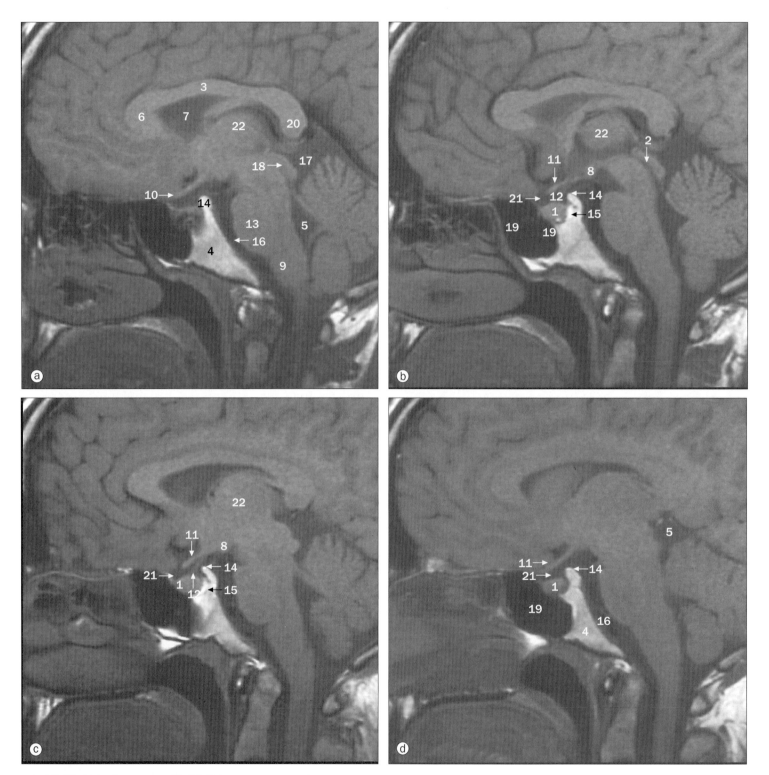

(a)–(d) Pituitary fossa, sagittal MR images.

1 Anterior pituitary gland	**9** Medulla oblongata	**17** Quadrigeminal cistern
2 Aqueduct of Sylvius	**10** Optic chiasma in suprasellar cistern	**18** Quadrigeminal plate of midbrain
3 Body of corpus callosum	**11** Optic tract	**19** Sphenoidal sinus
4 Fat in marrow of clivus	**12** Pituitary stalk	**20** Splenium of corpus callosum
5 Fourth ventricle	**13** Pons	**21** Suprasellar cistern
6 Genu of corpus callosum	**14** Posterior clinoid process	**22** Thalamus
7 Lateral ventricle	**15** Posterior pituitary gland	
8 Mammillary body	**16** Prepontine cistern	

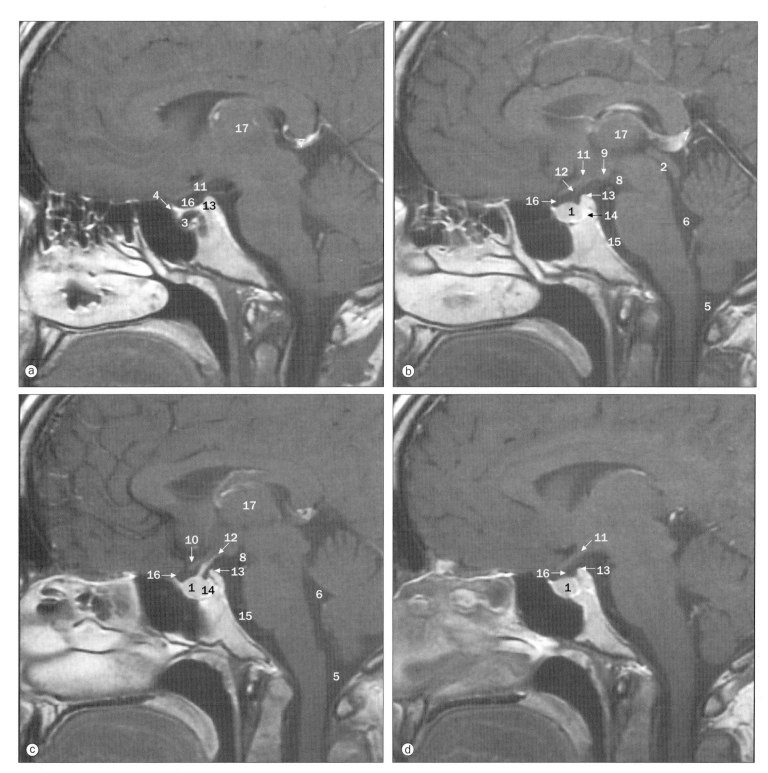

(a)–(d) Pituitary fossa, sagittal MR images, post gadolinium.

1 Anterior pituitary gland	**10** Optic chiasma
2 Aqueduct of Sylvius	**11** Optic tract
3 Cavernous portion of internal carotid artery	**12** Pituitary stalk
4 Cavernous sinus	**13** Posterior clinoid process
5 Cisterna magna (cerebellomedullary cistern)	**14** Posterior pituitary gland
6 Fourth ventricle	**15** Prepontine cistern
7 Great cerebral vein of Galen	**16** Suprasellar cistern
8 Interpeduncular cistern	**17** Thalamus
9 Mammillary body	

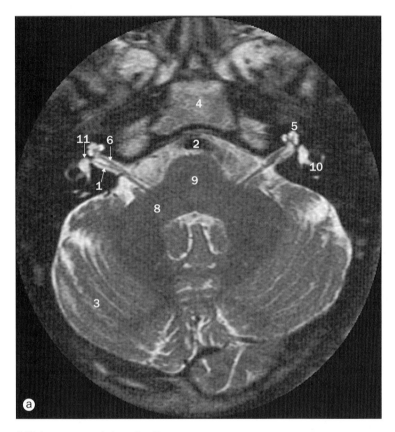

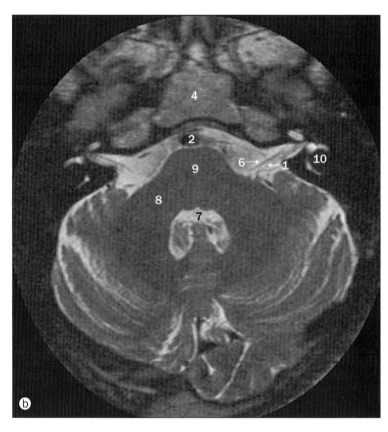

MR images, axial projection.

1 Auditory nerve (8th cranial nerve)
2 Basilar artery
3 Cerebellar hemisphere
4 Clivus
5 Cochlea
6 Facial nerve (7th cranial nerve)
7 Fourth ventricle
8 Middle cerebellar penduncle
9 Pons
10 Semi-circular canals
11 Vestibule

2 Vertebral column and spinal cord

(a) Cervical spine, anteroposterior projection.

(b) Dried cervical vertebra, anteroposterior projection.

1 Body of vertebra
2 Inferior articular process (facet)
3 Intertubercular lamella of transverse process
4 Posterior tubercle of transverse process
5 Posterolateral lip (uncus)
6 Region of vocal cords
7 Spinous process
8 Superior articular process (facet)
9 Trachea

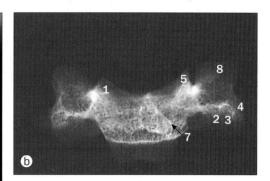
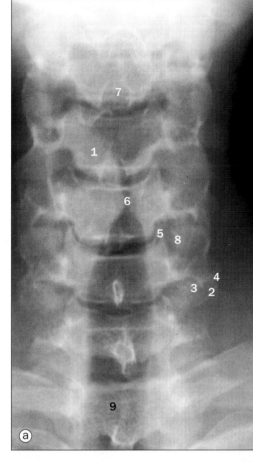

(c) Cervical spine, lateral projection; (d) dried atlas (first cervical vertebra), lateral projection; (e) dried axis (second cervical vertebra), lateral projection; (f) dried fourth cervical vertebra, lateral projection.

1 Anterior arch of atlas (first cervical vertebra)
2 Anterior tubercle of transverse process of fourth cervical vertebra
3 Body of axis (second cervical vertebra)
4 Inferior articular process (facet) of fourth cervical vertebra
5 Odontoid process (dens) of axis (second cervical vertebra)
6 Posterior arch of atlas (first cervical vertebra)
7 Posterior tubercle of atlas (first cervical vertebra)
8 Posterior tubercle of transverse process of fourth cervical vertebra
9 Spinous process of atlas (first cervical vertebra)
10 Spinous process of axis (second cervical vertebra)
11 Spinous process of fourth cervical vertebra
12 Superior articular process (facet) of fourth cervical vertebra

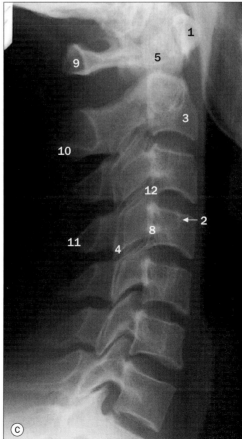
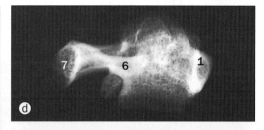
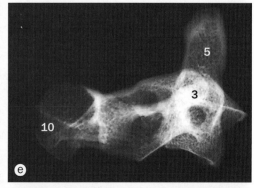
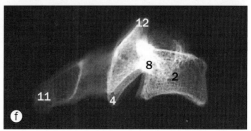

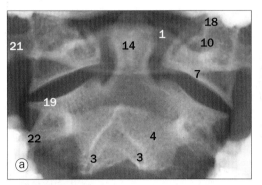

(a)

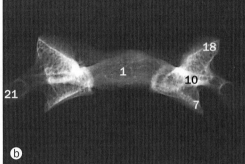

(b)

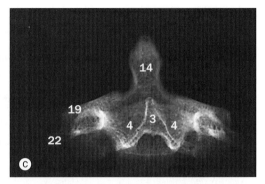

(c)

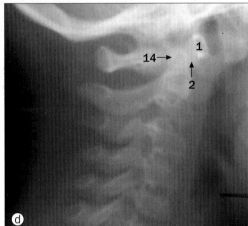

(d)

(a) Atlas (first cervical vertebra) and axis (second cervical vertebra), 'open mouth' anteroposterior projection.
(b) Dried atlas (first cervical vertebra), anteroposterior projection.
(c) Dried axis (second cervical vertebra), anteroposterior projection.
(d) Cervical spine of a 3-year-old child, lateral projection.
· The apparent widening of the atlanto-axial joint (2) is a normal feature at this age.
(e) Cervical spine, oblique projection.
(f) Line drawing of (e).

 1 Anterior arch of atlas (first cervical vertebra)
 2 Atlanto-axial joint of axis (second cervical vertebra)
 3 Bifid spinous process of axis (second cervical vertebra)
 4 Body of axis (second cervical vertebra)
 5 Body of fifth cervical vertebra
 6 Hyoid bone
 7 Inferior articular process (facet) of atlas (first cervical vertebra)
 8 Intervertebral foramen
 9 Lamina of fifth cervical vertebra
10 Lateral mass of atlas (first cervical vertebra)

11 Left first rib
12 Mandible
13 Occipital bone
14 Odontoid process (dens) of axis (second cervical vertebra)
15 Posterior tubercle of transverse process of fifth cervical vertebra
16 Posterolateral lip (uncus) of fifth cervical vertebra
17 Right first rib
18 Spinous process of fifth cervical vertebra
19 Superior articular process (facet) of atlas (first cervical vertebra)
20 Superior articular process (facet) of axis (second cervical vertebra)
21 Trachea
22 Transverse process of atlas (first cervical vertebra)
23 Transverse process of axis (second cervical vertebra)
24 Transverse process of fifth cervical vertebra

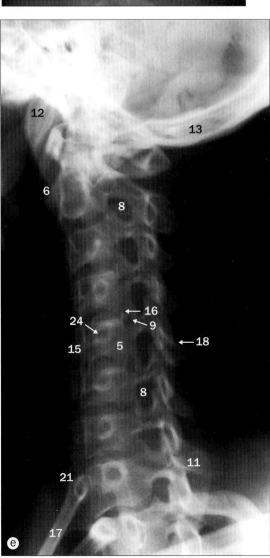

(e)

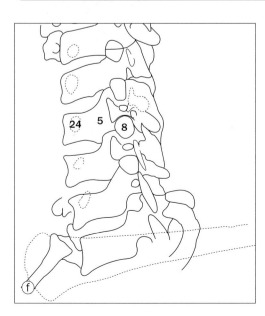

(f)

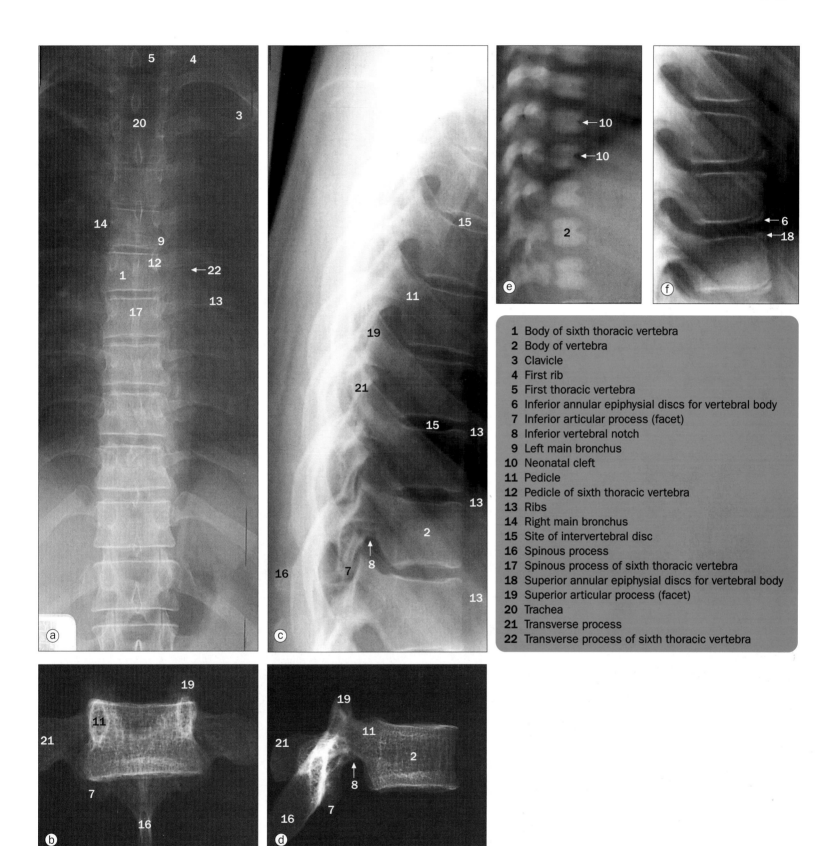

1 Body of sixth thoracic vertebra
2 Body of vertebra
3 Clavicle
4 First rib
5 First thoracic vertebra
6 Inferior annular epiphysial discs for vertebral body
7 Inferior articular process (facet)
8 Inferior vertebral notch
9 Left main bronchus
10 Neonatal cleft
11 Pedicle
12 Pedicle of sixth thoracic vertebra
13 Ribs
14 Right main bronchus
15 Site of intervertebral disc
16 Spinous process
17 Spinous process of sixth thoracic vertebra
18 Superior annular epiphysial discs for vertebral body
19 Superior articular process (facet)
20 Trachea
21 Transverse process
22 Transverse process of sixth thoracic vertebra

(a) Thoracic spine, anteroposterior projection.

(b) Dried thoracic vertebra, anteroposterior projection.

(c) Thoracic spine, lateral projection.

(d) Dried sixth thoracic vertebra, lateral projection.

Thoracic spine, (e) of a 7-day-old neonate, (f) of a 12-year-old child, lateral projections.

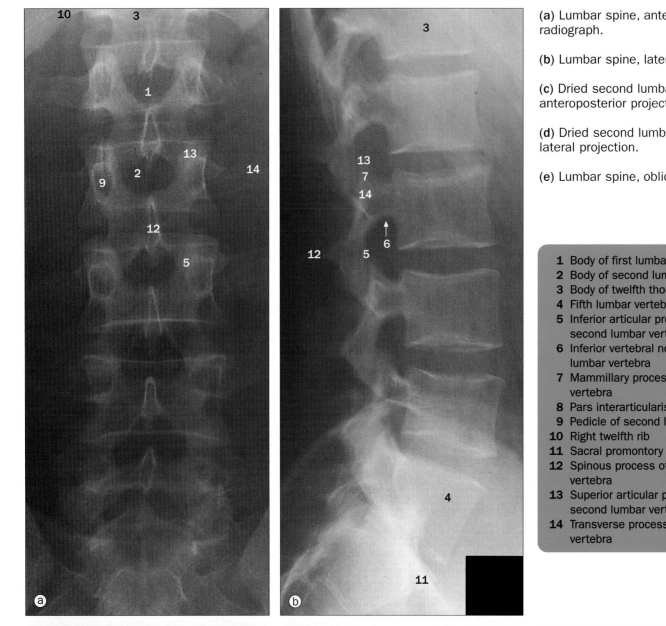

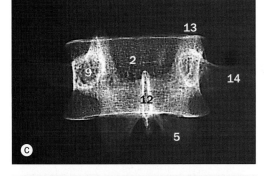

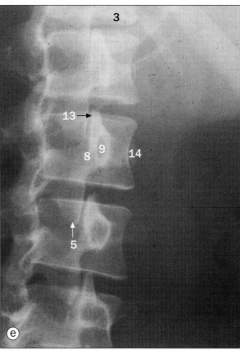

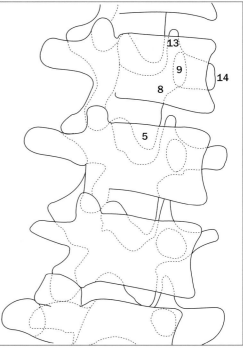

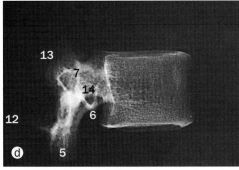

(a) Lumbar spine, anteroposterior radiograph.

(b) Lumbar spine, lateral projection.

(c) Dried second lumbar vertebra, anteroposterior projection.

(d) Dried second lumbar vertebra, lateral projection.

(e) Lumbar spine, oblique projection.

1 Body of first lumbar vertebra
2 Body of second lumbar vertebra
3 Body of twelfth thoracic vertebra
4 Fifth lumbar vertebra
5 Inferior articular process (facet) of second lumbar vertebra
6 Inferior vertebral notch of second lumbar vertebra
7 Mammillary process of second lumbar vertebra
8 Pars interarticularis
9 Pedicle of second lumbar vertebra
10 Right twelfth rib
11 Sacral promontory
12 Spinous process of second lumbar vertebra
13 Superior articular process (facet) of second lumbar vertebra
14 Transverse process of second lumbar vertebra

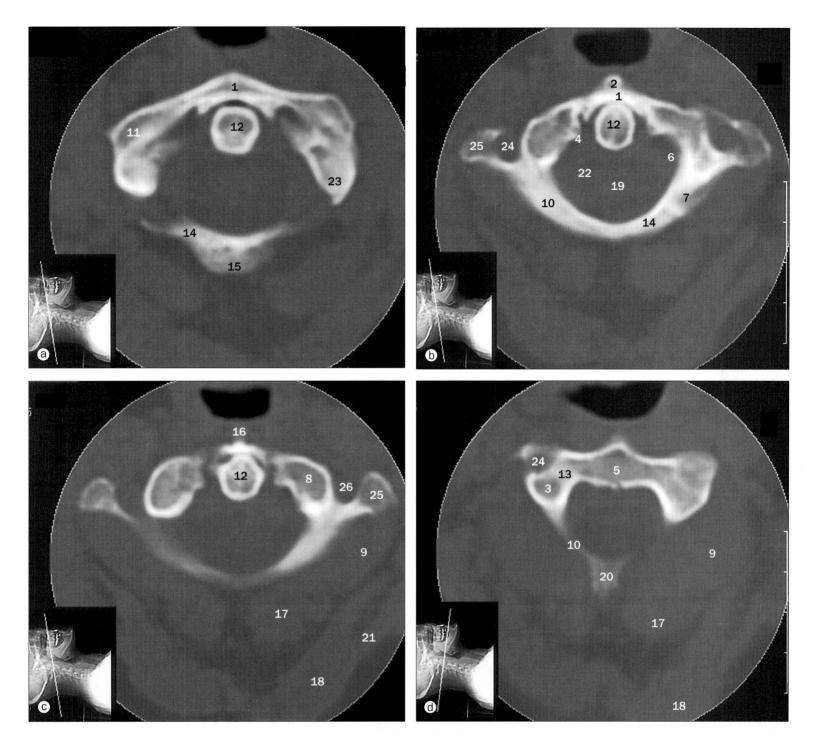

(a)–(d) Cervical spine, axial CT images at the level of the atlas (first cervical vertebra).

1 Anterior arch of atlas (first cervical vertebra)
2 Anterior tubercle of atlas
3 Articular pillar
4 Attachment of transverse ligament
5 Body of axis (second cervical vertebra)
6 Epidural space
7 Groove for vertebral artery
8 Inferior articular process (facet)
9 Inferior oblique muscle
10 Lamina
11 Lateral mass of atlas (first cervical vertebra)
12 Odontoid process (dens) of axis (second cervical vertebra)
13 Pedicle
14 Posterior arch of atlas (first cervical vertebra)
15 Posterior tubercle of atlas (first cervical vertebra)
16 Prevertebral soft tissue
17 Rectus capitis muscle
18 Semispinalis capitis muscle
19 Spinal cord
20 Spinous process of axis
21 Splenius capitis muscle
22 Subarachnoid space
23 Superior articular process (facet) of atlas (first cervical vertebra)
24 Transverse foramen
25 Transverse process
26 Vertebral artery in transverse foramen

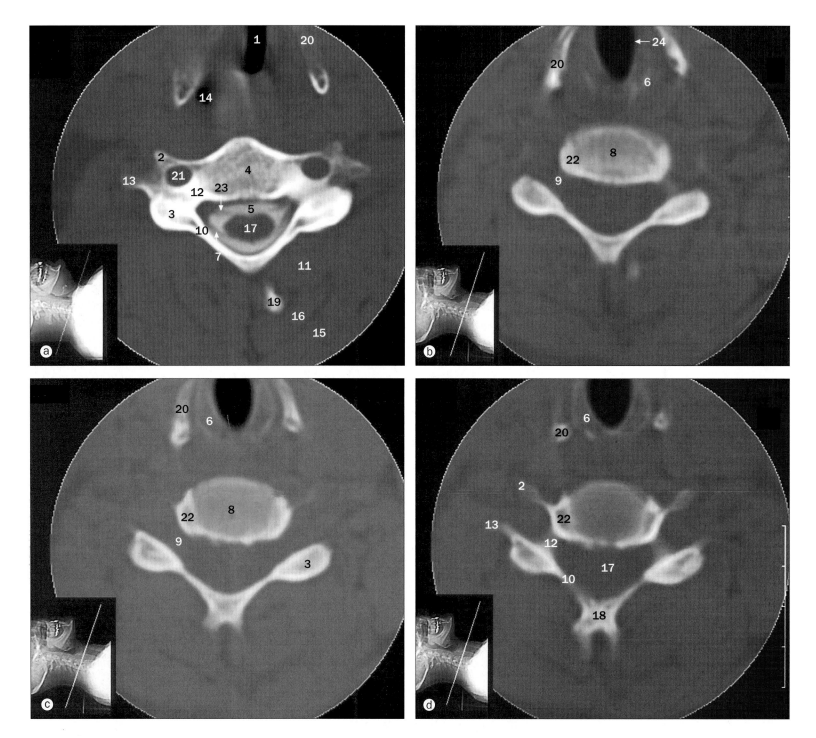

(a)–(d) Cervical spine, axial CT images at the level of the fifth and sixth cervical vertebrae.

1 Airway at level of vocal cord	**9** Intervertebral foramen	**18** Spinous process
2 Anterior tubercle	**10** Lamina	**19** Spinous process of fourth cervical vertebra
3 Articular pillar	**11** Multifidus muscle	**20** Thyroid cartilage
4 Body of fifth cervical vertebra	**12** Pedicle	**21** Transverse foramen
5 Contrast medium in subarachnoid space	**13** Posterior tubercle	**22** Uncinate process
6 Cricoid cartilage	**14** Pyriform sinus	**23** Ventral ramus
7 Dorsal ramus	**15** Semispinalis capitis muscle	**24** Vocal cord
8 Intervertebral disc (between fifth and sixth cervical vertebra)	**16** Semispinalis cervicis muscle	
	17 Spinal cord	

(a) and (b) Cervical spine, axial MR images.

1 Anterior longitudinal ligament and cortical bone
2 Body of vertebra
3 Cerebrospinal fluid in subarachnoid space
4 Common carotid artery
5 Dorsal ramus
6 Dorsal root ganglion
7 Epidural fat
8 Grey matter of cervical spinal cord
9 Inferior articular process (facet)
10 Internal jugular vein
11 Intervertebral foramen
12 Lamina
13 Levator scapulae muscle
14 Ligamentum flavum
15 Longus cervicis muscle
16 Multifidus muscle
17 Oesophagus
18 Posterior longitudinal ligament and cortical bone
19 Semispinalis capitis muscle
20 Spinous process
21 Splenius capitis muscle
22 Sternocleidomastoid muscle
23 Superior articular process (facet)
24 Thyroid gland
25 Trachea
26 Trapezius muscle
27 Ventral ramus
28 Vertebral artery in transverse foramen
29 White matter of cervical spinal cord
30 Zygapophysial (facet joint)

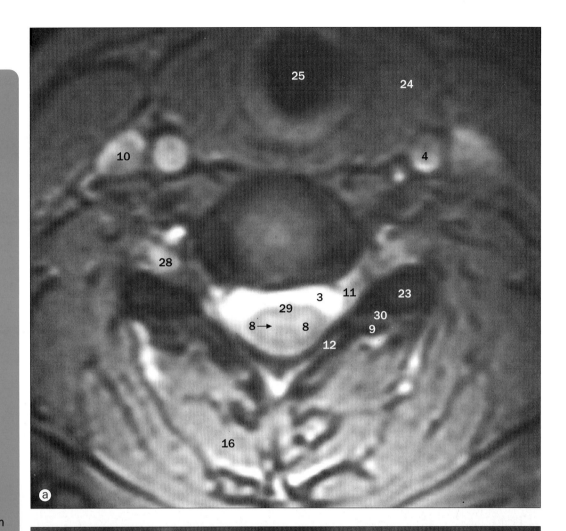

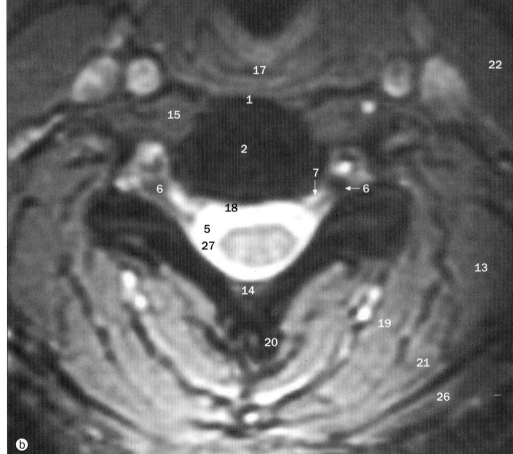

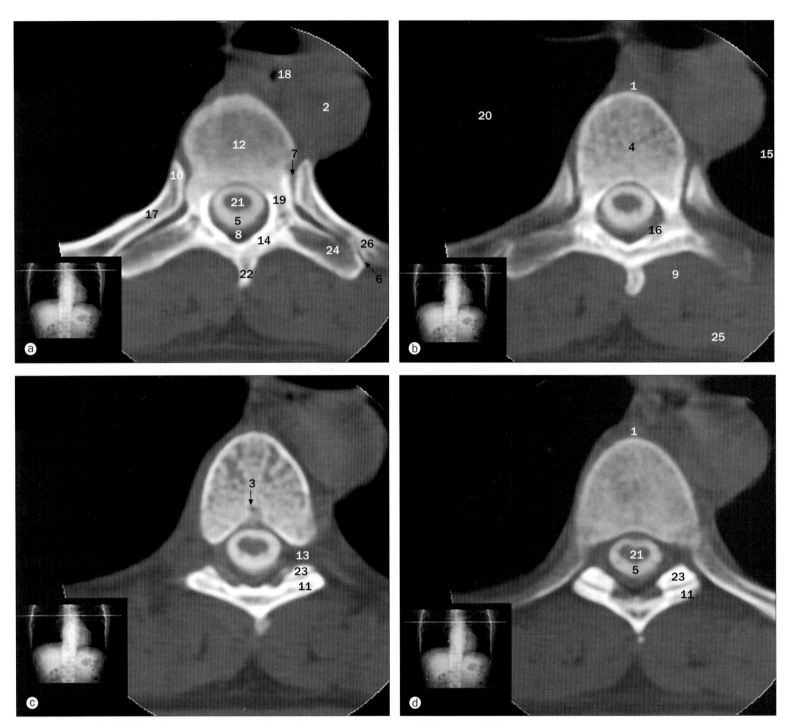

(a)–(d) Thoracic spine, axial CT images at the level of the sixth thoracic vertebra (with intrathecal contrast medium).

1 Anterior longitudinal ligament	**11** Inferior articular process (facet) of sixth thoracic vertebra	**19** Pedicle
2 Aorta		**20** Right lung
3 Basivertebral veins	**12** Intervertebral disc (between fifth and sixth thoracic vertebrae)	**21** Spinal cord
4 Body of sixth thoracic vertebra		**22** Spinous process
5 Contrast medium in subarachnoid space	**13** Intervertebral foramen	**23** Superior articular process (facet) of seventh thoracic vertebra
6 Costotransverse joint	**14** Lamina	
7 Costovertebral joint	**15** Left lung	**24** Transverse process
8 Epidural space	**16** Ligamentum flavum	**25** Trapezius muscle
9 Erector spinae muscles	**17** Neck of rib	**26** Tubercle of rib
10 Head of rib	**18** Oesophagus	

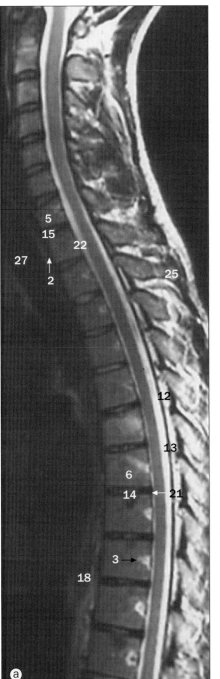

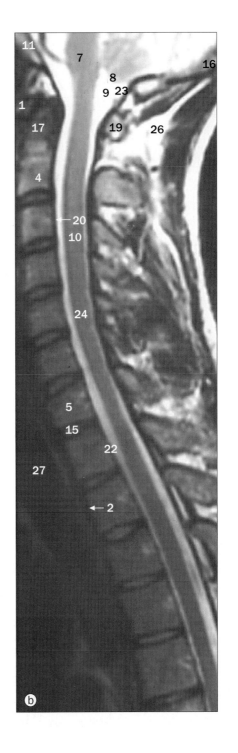

Spinal cord, (a) and (b) sagittal MR images.

1 Anterior arch of atlas (first cervical vertebra)
2 Anterior longitudinal ligament and cortical bone
3 Basivertebral vein
4 Body of axis (second cervical vertebra)
5 Body of seventh cervical vertebra
6 Body of seventh thoracic vertebra
7 Brainstem
8 Cerebellar tonsil
9 Cerebrospinal fluid in subarachnoid space
10 Cervical expansion
11 Clivus
12 Epidural fat
13 Ligamentum flavum
14 Nucleus pulposus of intervertebral disc
   (between seventh and eighth thoracic vertebrae)
15 Nucleus pulposus of intervertebral disc
   (between seventh cervical and first thoracic vertebrae)
16 Occipital bone
17 Odontoid process (dens)
18 Oesophagus
19 Posterior arch of atlas (first cervical vertebra)
20 Posterior longitudinal ligament
21 Posterior longitudinal ligament and annulus fibrosus
22 Posterior longitudinal ligament and cortical bone
23 Posterior margin of foramen magnum
24 Spinal cord
25 Spinous process
26 Suboccipital fat
27 Trachea

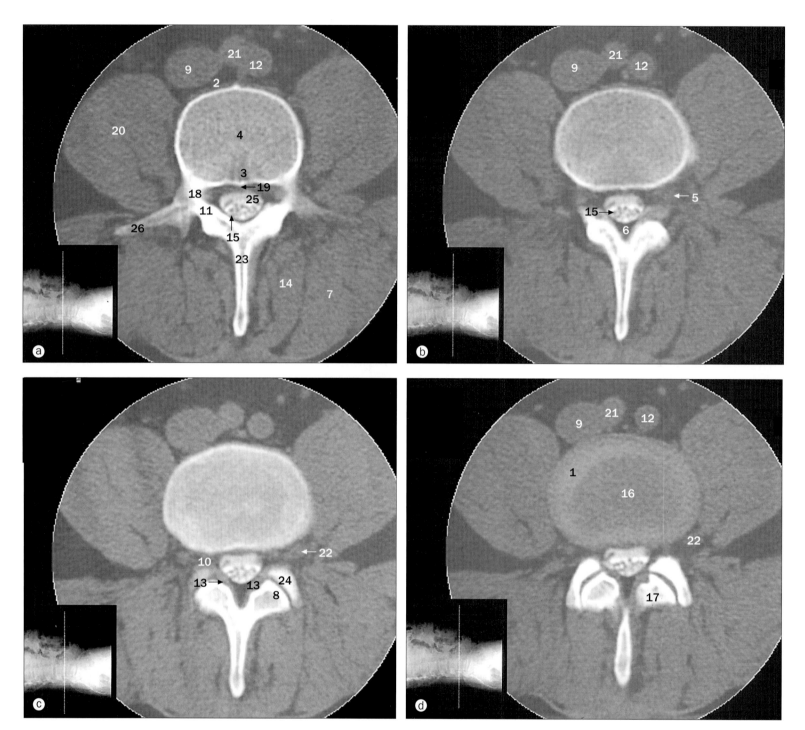

(a)–(d) Lumbar spine, axial CT images at the level of the fourth and fifth lumbar vertebrae (with intrathecal contrast medium).

Multiple thin (5 mm) sections are taken parallel to the disc space. Lumbar epidural fat provides contrast around the theca and exiting nerve roots, and the posterior aspect of the disc.

1 Annulus fibrosus of intervertebral disc	**10** Intervertebral foramen (between fourth and fifth lumbar vertebrae)	**19** Posterior longitudinal ligament
2 Anterior longitudinal ligament		**20** Psoas muscle
3 Basivertebral veins	**11** Lamina	**21** Right common iliac artery
4 Body of fourth lumbar vertebra	**12** Left common iliac artery	**22** Root of fourth lumbar nerve
5 Dorsal root ganglion of fourth lumbar nerve	**13** Ligamentum flavum	**23** Spinous process of fourth lumbar vertebra
6 Epidural fat	**14** Multifidus muscle	
7 Erector spinae muscle	**15** Nerve roots of cauda equina	**24** Superior articular process (facet) of fifth lumbar vertebrae
8 Inferior articular process (facet) of fourth lumbar vertebra	**16** Nucleus pulposus of intervertebral disc	
	17 Pars interarticularis	**25** Thecal sac
9 Inferior vena cava	**18** Pedicle	**26** Transverse process

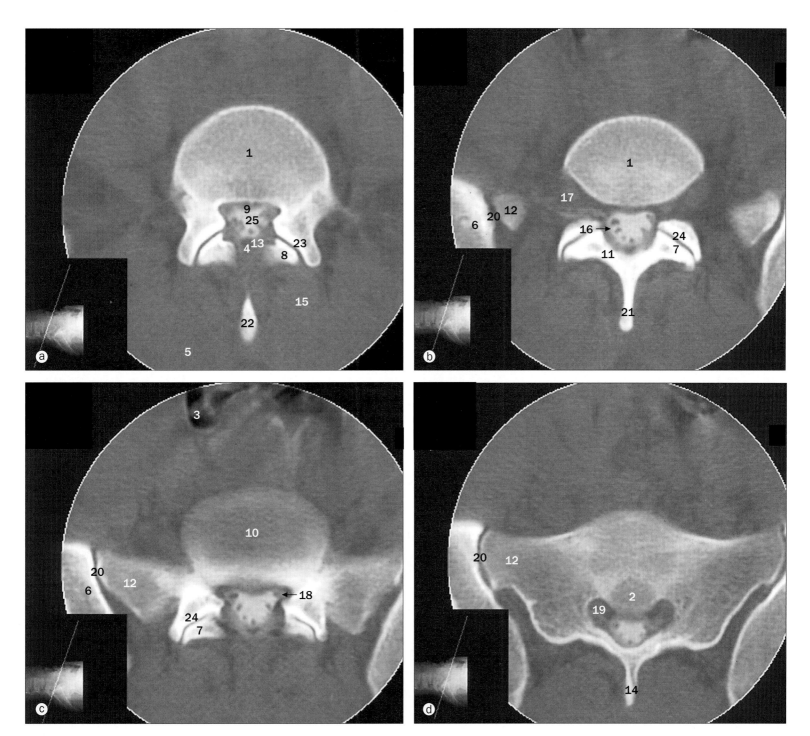

(a)–(d) Lumbar spine, axial CT images at the level of the lumbrosacral junction (with intrathecal contrast medium).

1	Body of fifth lumbar vertebra	**9**	Internal vertebral veins
2	Body of sacrum	**10**	Intervertebral disc (fifth lumbar/first sacral vertebra)
3	Bowel gas		
4	Epidural fat	**11**	Lamina
5	Erector spinae muscle	**12**	Lateral part (ala) of sacrum
6	Ilium	**13**	Ligamentum flavum
7	Inferior articular process (facet) of fifth lumbar vertebra	**14**	Median sacral crest
		15	Multifidus muscle
8	Inferior articular process (facet) of fourth lumbar vertebra	**16**	Nerve roots of cauda equina
		17	Root of fifth lumbar nerve

18	Root of first sacral nerve
19	Sacral foramina
20	Sacro-iliac joint
21	Spinous process of fifth lumbar vertebra
22	Spinous process of fourth lumbar vertebra
23	Superior articular process (facet) of fifth lumbar vertebra
24	Superior articular process (facet) of first sacral vertebra
25	Thecal sac

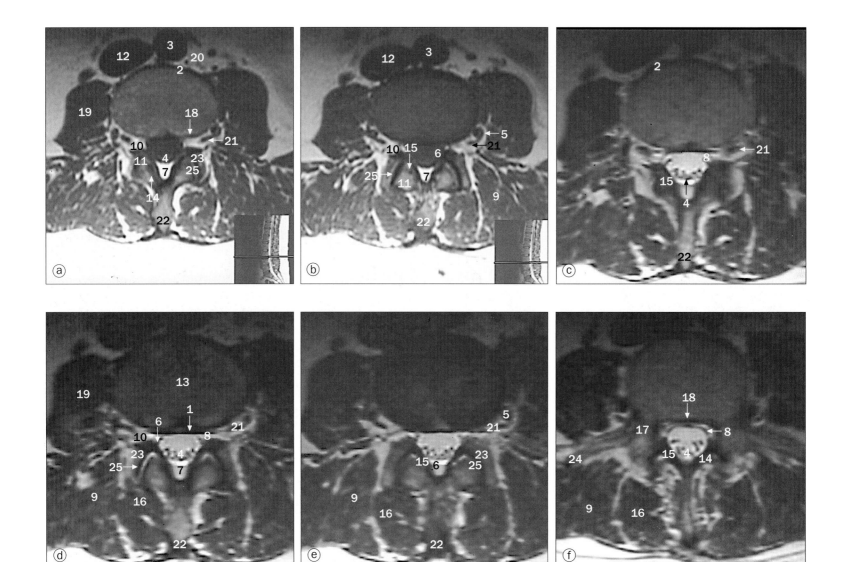

(a)–(f) Lumbar spine, axial MR images.

1 Annulus fibrosus and posterior longitudinal ligament	**14** Lamina
2 Anterior longitudinal ligament and cortical bone	**15** Ligamentum flavum
3 Aorta	**16** Multifidus muscle
4 Cauda equina in lumbar thecal sac	**17** Pedicle
5 Dorsal root ganglion	**18** Posterior longitudinal ligament
6 Dura	**19** Psoas muscle
7 Epidural fat in epidural space	**20** Retroperitoneal fat
8 Epidural veins in epidural space	**21** Spinal nerve root
9 Erector spinae muscles	**22** Spinous process
10 Fat in intervertebral foramen	**23** Superior articular process (facet)
11 Inferior articular process (facet)	**24** Transverse process
12 Inferior vena cava	**25** Zygapophysial (facet) joint
13 Intervertebral disc	

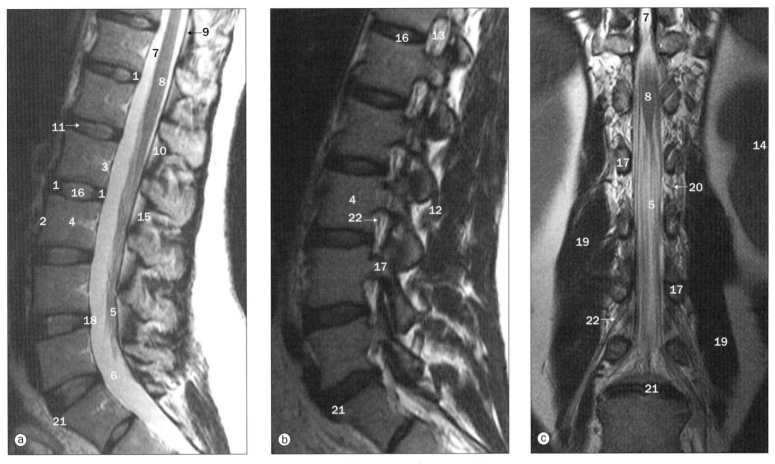

Lumbosacral spine, (a) sagittal MR image, (b) parasagittal MR image, (c) coronal MR image.

1 Annulus fibrosus	**12** Interspinous ligament and bursa
2 Anterior longitudinal ligament	**13** Intervertebral foramen
3 Basivertebral veins	**14** Kidney
4 Body of third lumbar vertebra	**15** Ligamentum flavum
5 Cauda equina	**16** Nucleus pulposus
6 Caudal lumbar thecal sac	**17** Pedicle
7 Cerebrospinal fluid	**18** Posterior longitudinal ligament and annulus fibrosus
8 Conus medullaris	**19** Psoas muscle
9 Epidural fat	**20** Radicular vessels
10 Epidural space (fat filled)	**21** Sacral promontory
11 Internuclear cleft	**22** Spinal nerve root in intervertebral foramen

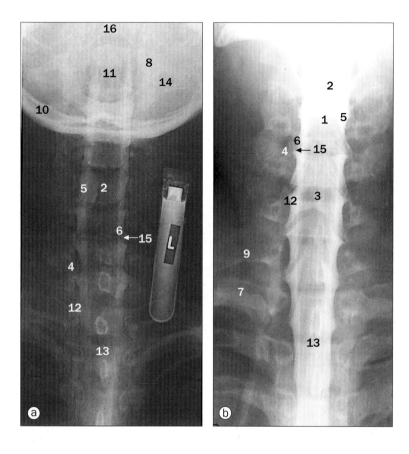

Cervical myelogram, (a) with the neck extended, (b) with the neck slightly flexed, anteroposterior projections.

Non-ionic water-soluble contrast medium is introduced into the lumbar subarachnoid space via a lumbar puncture. The patient is positioned prone, with the neck hyperextended, and strapped onto a tilting table. The contrast medium is then run up into the cervical region to demonstrate the cervical spinal cord and exiting nerve roots. There are eight cervical nerve roots: the roots of the eighth cervical nerve exit through the intervertebral foramina between the seventh cervical vertebra and the first thoracic vertebra. The normal cervical cord enlargement (3) (for the brachial plexus) extends from the third cervical vertebra to the second thoracic vertebra. It is maximal at the fifth cervical vertebra and should not be mistaken for an intramedullary lesion.

1 Anterior spinal artery
2 Cervical cord
3 Cervical cord enlargement
4 Cervical spinal nerve exiting through intervertebral foramen
5 Contrast medium in cervical subarachnoid space
6 Dorsal root of spinal nerve
7 First rib
8 Lateral mass of atlas (first cervical vertebra)
9 Normal large transverse process of seventh cervical vertebra
10 Occiput
11 Odontoid process (dens)
12 Root of eighth cervical nerve
13 Thoracic cord
14 Transverse foramen
15 Ventral root of spinal nerve
16 Vertebral artery

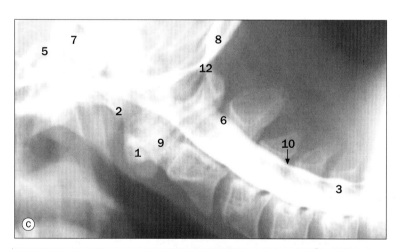

Cervical myelogram, (c) with the patient prone, (d) with the patient supine, lateral projections.

1 Anterior arch of atlas (first cervical vertebra)
2 Anterior rim of foramen magnum
3 Cervical cord
4 Cisterna magna (cerebellomedullary cistern)
5 Clivus
6 Contrast medium in cervical subarachnoid space
7 External acoustic meatus
8 Occiput
9 Odontoid (process) dens
10 Posterior indentation on theca from ligamentum flavum
11 Posterior inferior cerebellar artery
12 Posterior rim of foramen magnum
13 Posterior tubercle of atlas (first cervical vertebra)

Lumbar radiculogram, (a) lateral projection, (b) oblique projection, (c) anteroposterior projection.

Non-ionic water-soluble contrast medium is introduced into the lumbar subarachnoid space via a lumbar puncture. The nerve roots of the cauda equina are well demonstrated and exit through the intervertebral foramina. The nerve roots extending from the conus to the terminal thecal sac pass below the pedicle of the corresponding vertebra. The thecal sac terminates at the level of the first/second sacral vertebrae. The filum terminale may be seen. Tilting the prone patient slightly head down allows the contrast to flow cranially and outlines the conus and lower thoracic cord. The cord is uniform in size from the second to the tenth thoracic vertebra, at which point its second, smaller expansion (for the lumbosacral plexus) extends from the tenth thoracic vertebra to the level of the first lumbar vertebra. The conus medullaris usually terminates at the first/second lumbar vertebrae, but may be seen at a level above and below as a normal variant.

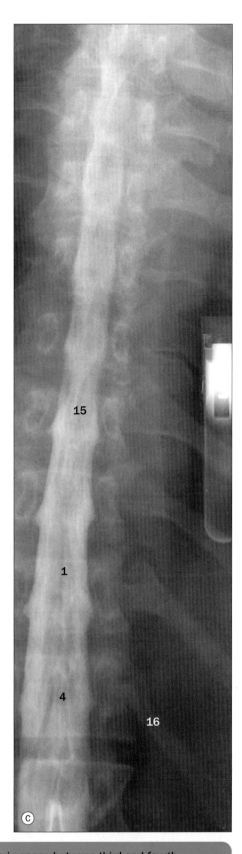

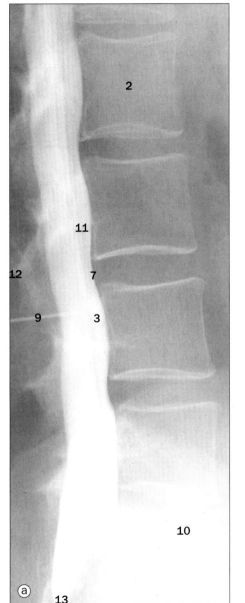

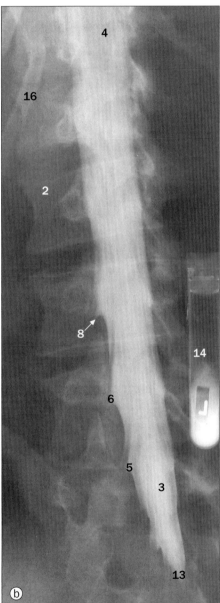

1 Anterior median fissure	**9** Lumbar puncture needle in space between third and fourth lumbar vertebrae
2 Body of second lumbar vertebra	**10** Sacral promontory
3 Contrast medium in subarachnoid space	**11** Spinal nerves within subarachnoid space (cauda equina)
4 Conus medullaris	**12** Spinous process of third lumbar vertebra
5 Fifth lumbar spinal nerve	**13** Terminal theca at first/second sacral vertebra
6 Fourth lumbar spinal nerve	**14** Test tube containing contrast medium to indicate tilt of patient
7 Intervertebral disc indentations in anterior thecal margin	**15** Thoracic cord
8 Lateral extension of subarachnoid space around spinal nerve roots	**16** Twelfth rib

(a) Subtracted lumbar venogram.
Since the advent of CT and MR imaging techniques, lumbar venography is rarely performed. However, the anatomy of the vertebral veins is optimally demonstrated by this technique. Venous drainage of the spinal cord is longitudinally arranged via plexi, which anastomose freely with the internal (6) and external (1 and 4) vertebral venous plexi, which also communicate (4 and 2). Note how the internal veins bend laterally at the level of the disc interspace and medially at the level of pedicles, where they unite via a connecting vein (2).

1 Ascending lumbar veins
2 Basivertebral veins
3 Catheter in common iliac vein
4 Intervertebral veins
5 Lateral sacral veins
6 Longitudinal vertebral venous plexi
7 Sacral venous plexus
8 Tip of catheter in intravertebral vein

(b) Spinal arteriogram.

1 Anterior spinal artery
2 Arteria radicularis magna (Adamkiewicz)
3 Normal transdural stenosis of the arteria radicularis magna
4 Selective catheterisation of left eleventh intercostal artery

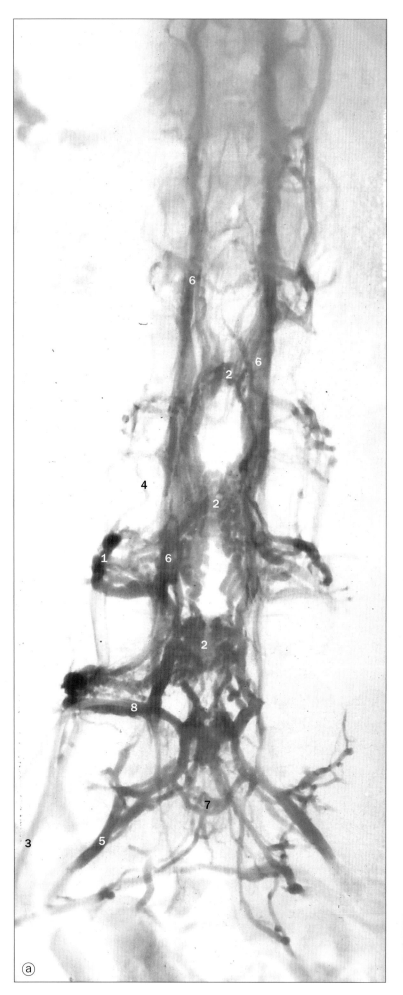

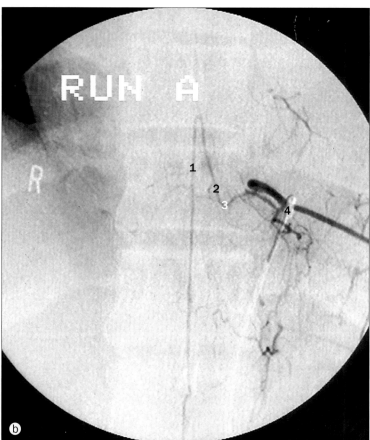

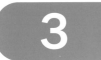

Upper limb

(a) Shoulder, anteroposterior radiograph.

1 Acromion of scapula
2 Anatomical neck
3 Clavicle
4 Coracoid process of scapula
5 Glenoid fossa of scapula
6 Greater tubercle (tuberosity) of humerus
7 Head of humerus
8 Intertubercular groove of humerus
9 Lesser tubercle (tuberosity) of humerus
10 Scapula
11 Surgical neck

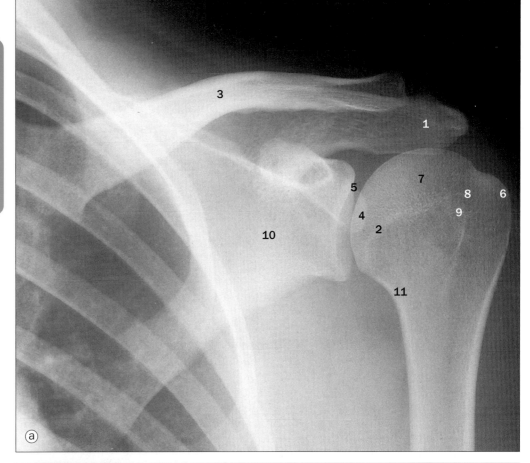

(b) Shoulder, axial (supero-inferior) projection.

1 Acromion of scapula
2 Clavicle
3 Coracoid process of scapula
4 Glenoid fossa of scapula
5 Greater tubercle (tuberosity) of humerus
6 Head of humerus
7 Intertubercular groove of humerus
8 Lesser tubercle (tuberosity) of humerus
9 Spine of scapula

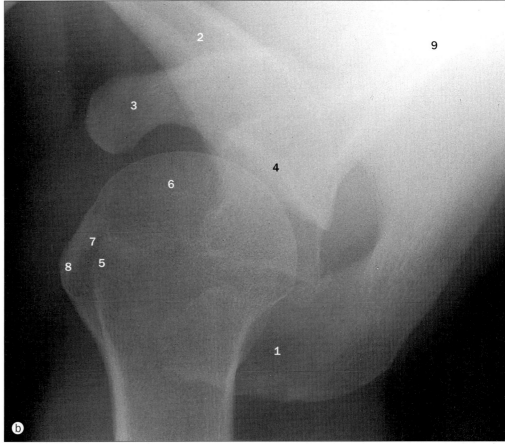

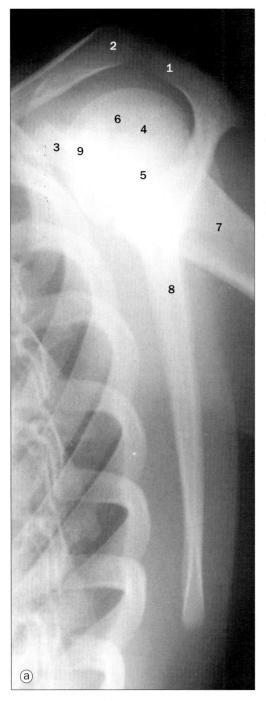

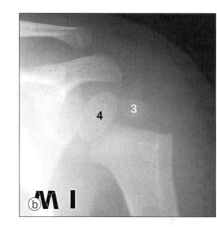

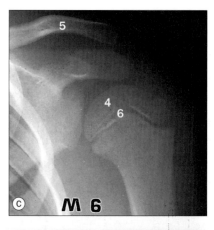

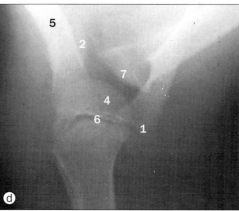

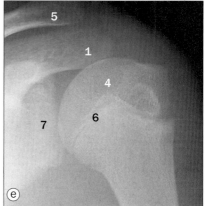

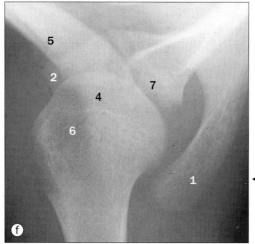

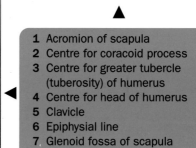

Shoulder, **(b)** (anteroposterior) of a 1-year-old child, **(c)** (anteroposterior) and **(d)** (axial) of a 6-year-old child, **(e)** (anteroposterior) and **(f)** (axial) of a 14-year-old child.

▲

1 Acromion of scapula
2 Centre for coracoid process
3 Centre for greater tubercle (tuberosity) of humerus
4 Centre for head of humerus
5 Clavicle
6 Epiphysial line
7 Glenoid fossa of scapula

(a) Scapula of a 14-year-old boy, lateral projection.

▲

1 Acromion
2 Clavicle
3 Coracoid process
4 Epiphysial line
5 Glenoid fossa
6 Head of humerus
7 Humerus
8 Lateral border of scapula
9 Spine of scapula

CLAVICLE (m)	Appears	Fused
Lateral end	5 wiu	20+ yrs
Medial end	15 yrs	20+ yrs
SCAPULA (c)		
Body	8 wiu	15 yrs
Coracoid	<1 yr	20 yrs
Coracoid base	Puberty	15–20 yrs
Acromion	Puberty	15–20 yrs

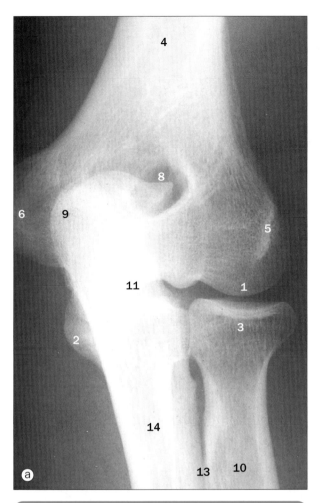

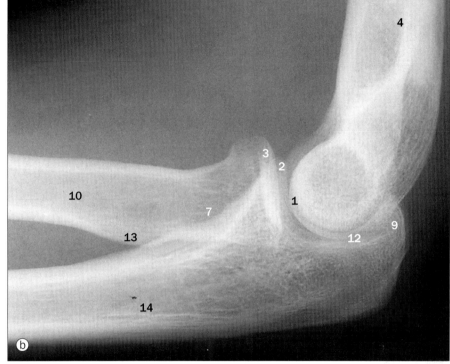

Elbow, (a) anteroposterior projection, (b) lateral projection, (c) axial projection.

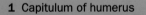

1 Capitulum of humerus
2 Coronoid process of ulna
3 Head of radius
4 Humerus
5 Lateral epicondyle of humerus
6 Medial epicondyle of humerus
7 Neck of radius
8 Olecranon fossa of humerus
9 Olecranon of ulna
10 Radius
11 Trochlea of humerus
12 Trochlear notch of ulna
13 Tuberosity of radius
14 Ulna

HUMERUS (c)	Appears	Fused
Shaft	8 wiu	15–20 yrs
Head	1–6 mths	15–20 yrs
Greater tubercle	6 mths–1 yr	15–20 yrs
Lesser tubercle	3–5 yrs	18–20 yrs
Capitulum	4 mths–1 yr	13–16 yrs
Medial trochlea	10 yrs	13–16 yrs
Medial epicondyle	3–6 yrs	13–16 yrs
Lateral epicondyle	9–12 yrs	13–16 yrs
RADIUS (c)		
Shaft	8 wiu	
Proximal	4–6 yrs	13–16 yrs
Distal	1 yr	16–18 yrs
ULNA (c)		
Shaft	8 wiu	
Proximal	8–10 yrs	13–15 yrs
Distal	5–7 yrs	16–18 yrs

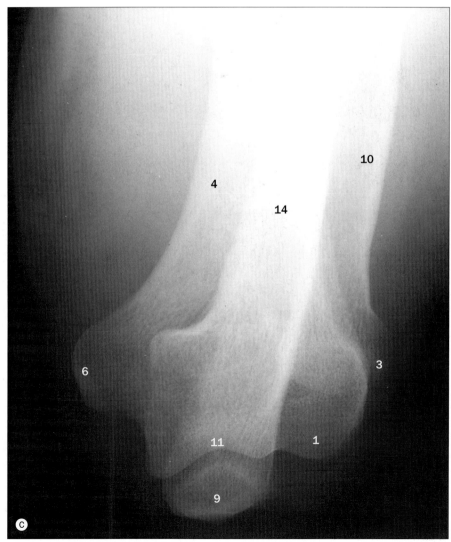

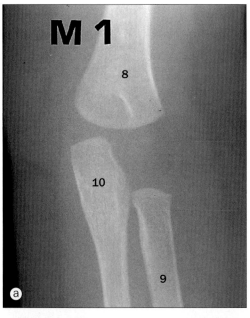

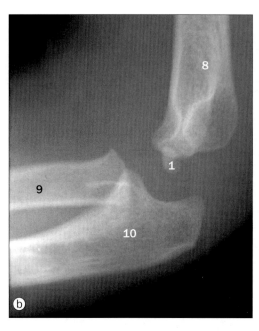

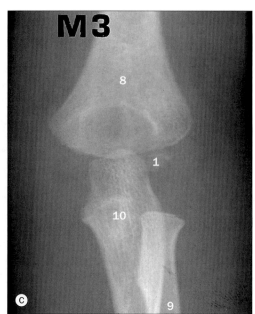

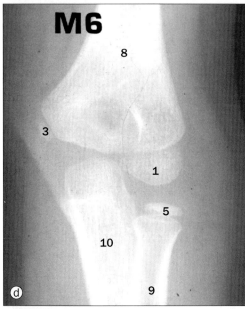

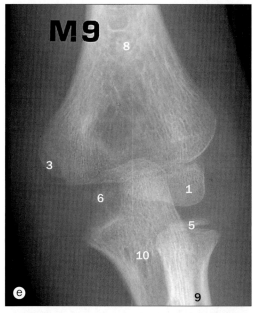

Elbow, **(a)** (anteroposterior) of a 1-year-old child, **(b)** (lateral) and **(c)** (anteroposterior) of a 3-year-old child, **(d)** (anteroposterior) of a 6-year-old child, **(e)** (anteroposterior) of a 9-year-old child, **(f)** (lateral) of an 11-year-old child, **(g)** (lateral) and **(h)** (anteroposterior) of a 14-year-old child, to illustrate centres of ossification.

1 Centre for capitulum
2 Centre for lateral epicondyle
3 Centre for medial epicondyle
4 Centre for olecranon
5 Centre for radial head
6 Centre for trochlea
7 Epiphysial line
8 Humerus
9 Radius
10 Ulna

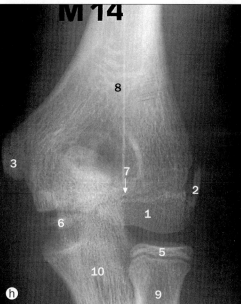

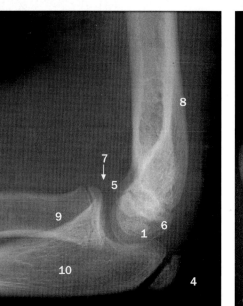

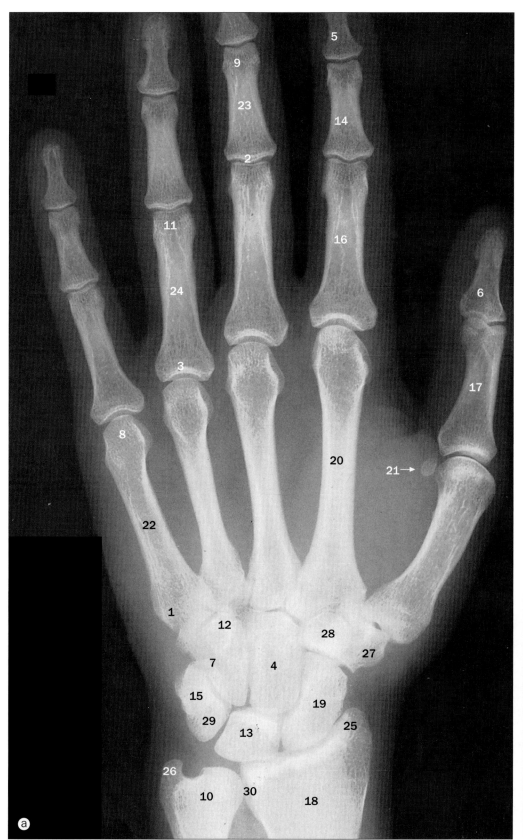

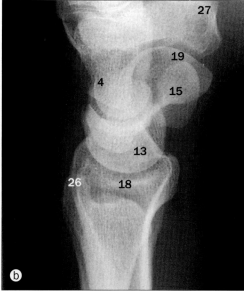

1	Base of fifth metacarpal
2	Base of middle phalanx of middle finger
3	Base of proximal phalanx of ring finger
4	Capitate
5	Distal phalanx of index finger
6	Distal phalanx of thumb
7	Hamate
8	Head of fifth metacarpal
9	Head of middle phalanx of middle finger
10	Head of ulna
11	Head of proximal phalanx of ring finger
12	Hook of hamate
13	Lunate
14	Middle phalanx of index finger
15	Pisiform
16	Proximal phalanx of index finger
17	Proximal phalanx of thumb
18	Radius
19	Scaphoid
20	Second metacarpal
21	Sesamoid bone
22	Shaft of fifth metacarpal
23	Shaft of middle phalanx of middle finger
24	Shaft of proximal phalanx of ring finger
25	Styloid process of radius
26	Styloid process of ulna
27	Trapezium
28	Trapezoid
29	Triquetral
30	Ulnar notch of radius

• There are often two sesamoids (21), present in the flexor pollicis brevis and adductor pollicis muscles.

(a) Bones of the hand, dorsopalmar projection.

(b) Bones of the wrist, lateral projection.

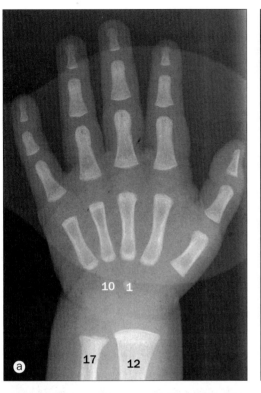

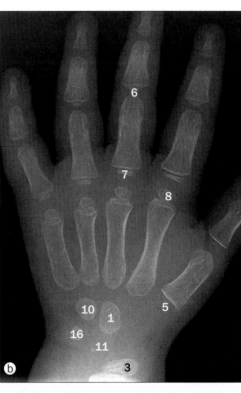

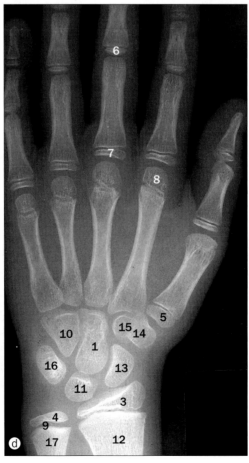

Bones of the hand (dorsopalmar projections), (a) of a 3-month-old boy, (b) of a 3-year-old boy, (c) of a 6-year-old boy, (d) of an 11-year-old boy, to illustrate centres of ossification.

CARPUS (c)	Appears	Fused
Capitate	1–3 mths	
Hamate	2–4 mths	
Triquetral	2–3 yrs	
Lunate	2–4 yrs	
Scaphoid	4–6 yrs	
Trapezium	4–6 yrs	
Trapezoid	4–6 yrs	
Pisiform (sesamoid)	8–12 yrs	
METACARPALS (c)		
Shaft	9 wiu	
Head	1–2 yrs	14–19 yrs
PHALANGES (c)		
Shaft	8–12 wiu	
Base	1–3 yrs	14–18 yrs

1 Capitate
2 Centre for distal phalanx of middle finger
3 Centre for distal radius
4 Centre for distal ulna
5 Centre for first metacarpal
6 Centre for middle phalanx of middle finger
7 Centre for proximal phalanx of middle finger
8 Centre for second metacarpal (applies to second to fifth metacarpals)
9 Epiphysial line
10 Hamate
11 Lunate
12 Radius
13 Scaphoid
14 Trapezium
15 Trapezoid
16 Triquetral
17 Ulna

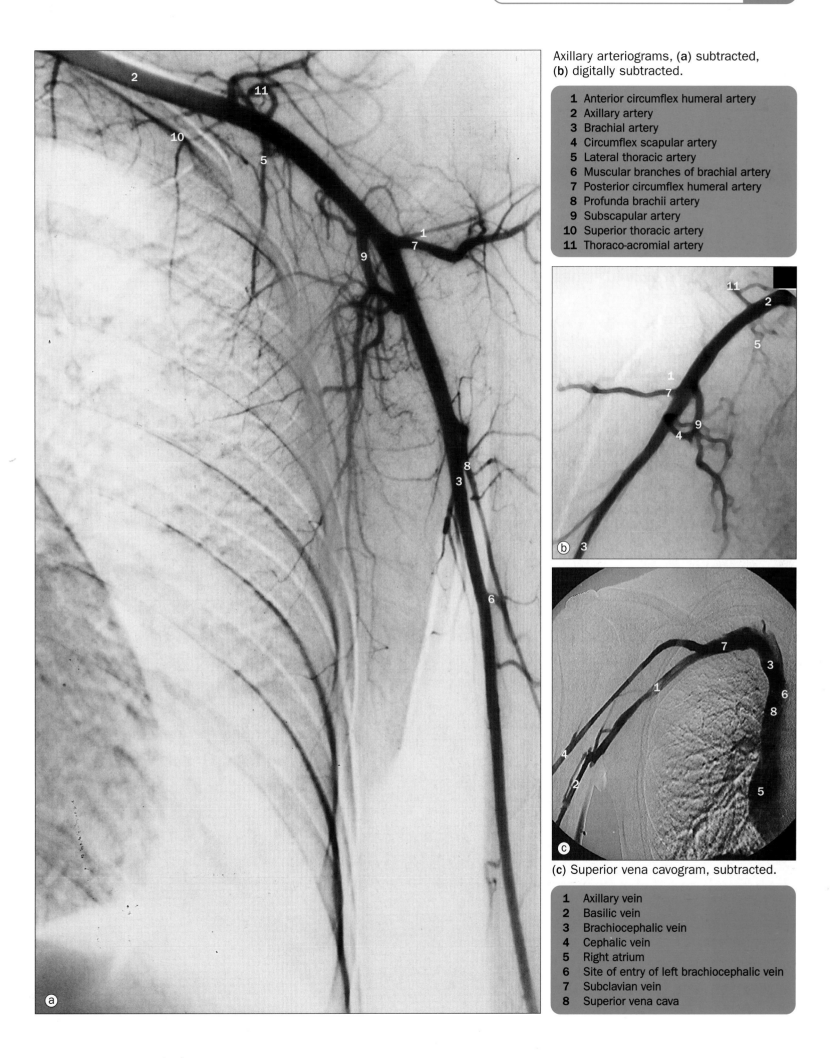

Axillary arteriograms, (a) subtracted, (b) digitally subtracted.

1	Anterior circumflex humeral artery
2	Axillary artery
3	Brachial artery
4	Circumflex scapular artery
5	Lateral thoracic artery
6	Muscular branches of brachial artery
7	Posterior circumflex humeral artery
8	Profunda brachii artery
9	Subscapular artery
10	Superior thoracic artery
11	Thoraco-acromial artery

(c) Superior vena cavogram, subtracted.

1	Axillary vein
2	Basilic vein
3	Brachiocephalic vein
4	Cephalic vein
5	Right atrium
6	Site of entry of left brachiocephalic vein
7	Subclavian vein
8	Superior vena cava

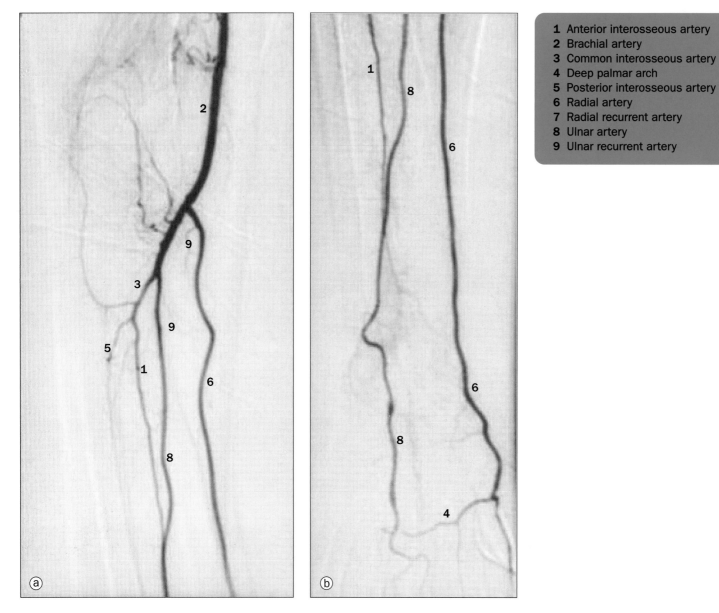

1 Anterior interosseous artery
2 Brachial artery
3 Common interosseous artery
4 Deep palmar arch
5 Posterior interosseous artery
6 Radial artery
7 Radial recurrent artery
8 Ulnar artery
9 Ulnar recurrent artery

Brachial arteriogram.

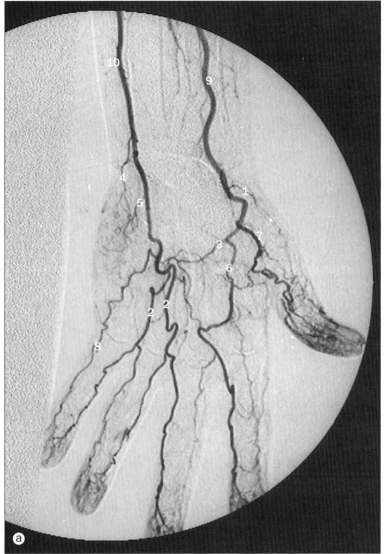

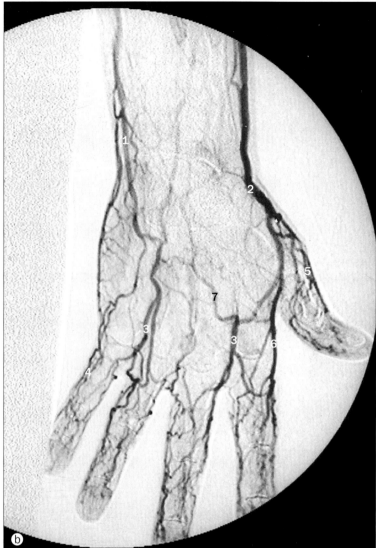

(a) Digitally subtracted hand arteriogram.
In this patient there is an incomplete superficial palmar arch.

(b) Venous phase of hand arteriogram.

 1 Artery to radial aspects of thumb
 2 Common palmar digital artery
 3 Deep palmar arch
 4 Deep palmar branch of ulnar artery
 5 Palmar carpal branch of ulnar artery
 6 Palmar metacarpal artery
 7 Princeps pollicis artery
 8 Proper palmar digital artery
 9 Radial artery
10 Ulnar artery

 1 Basilic vein
 2 Cephalic vein
 3 Common palmar digital vein
 4 Palmar digital vein
 5 Princeps pollicis vein
 6 Radialis indicis vein
 7 Superficial palmar venous arch

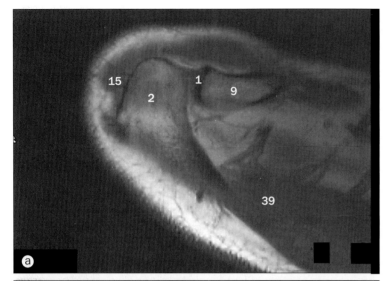

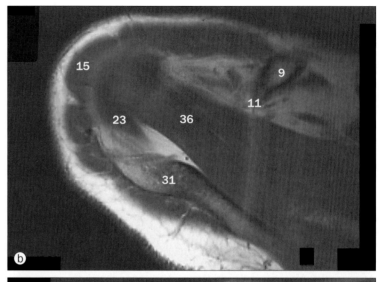

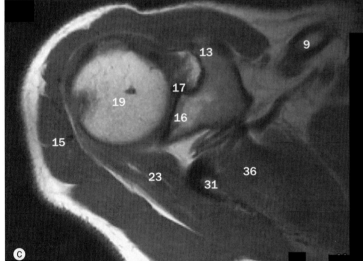

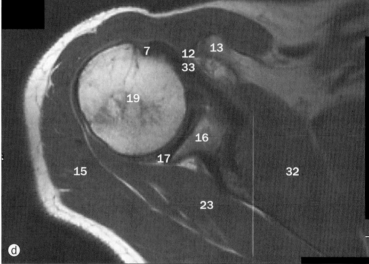

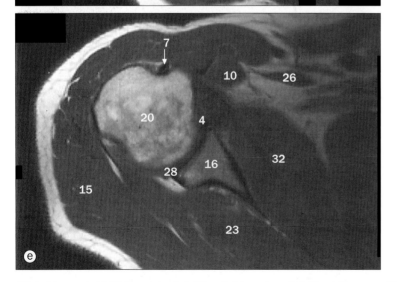

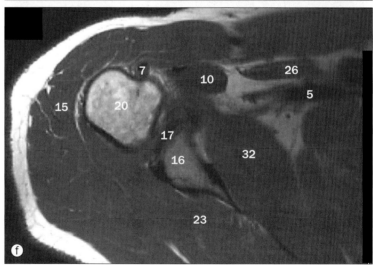

Shoulder, axial MR images, **(a)**–**(f)** axial images, **(g)**–**(l)** oblique sagittal images.

1 Acromioclavicular joint	**9** Clavicle	**17** Glenoid labrum
2 Acromion	**10** Coracobrachialis muscle	**18** Greater tuberosity
3 Anterior capsule of shoulder joint	**11** Coracoclavicular ligament	**19** Head of humerus
4 Anterior labrum	**12** Coracohumeral ligament	**20** Humerus
5 Axillary artery and vein	**13** Coracoid process	**21** Inferior glenohumeral ligament
6 Axillary recess	**14** Deltoid tendon	**22** Inferior labrum
7 Biceps brachii tendon	**15** Deltoid muscle	**23** Infraspinatus muscle
8 Biceps brachii tendon – long head	**16** Glenoid	**24** Infraspinatus tendon

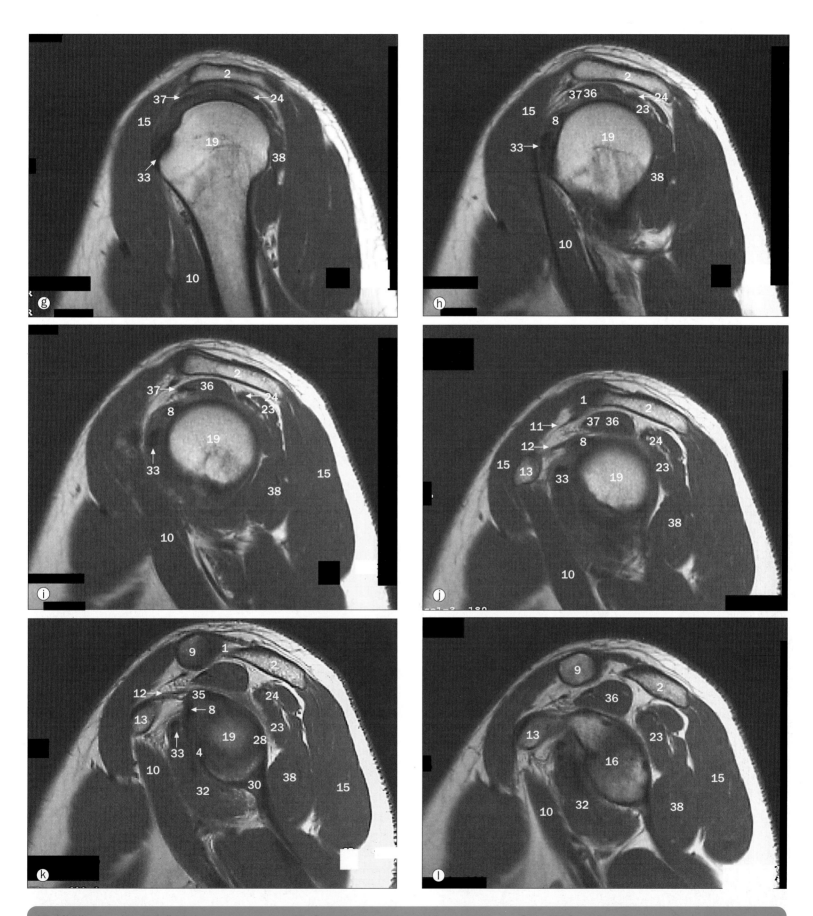

25	Middle glenohumeral ligament	30	Scapula	35	Superior labrum
26	Pectoralis minor muscle	31	Spine of scapula	36	Supraspinatus muscle
27	Posterior capsule of shoulder joint	32	Subscapularis muscle	37	Supraspinatus tendon
28	Posterior labrum	33	Subscapularis tendon	38	Teres minor muscle
29	Rotator cuff	34	Superior glenohumeral ligament	39	Trapezius muscle

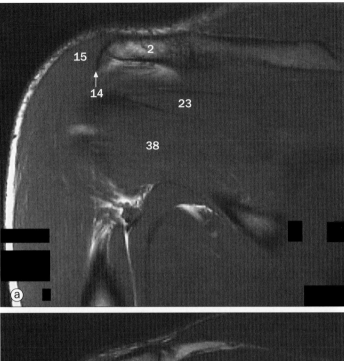

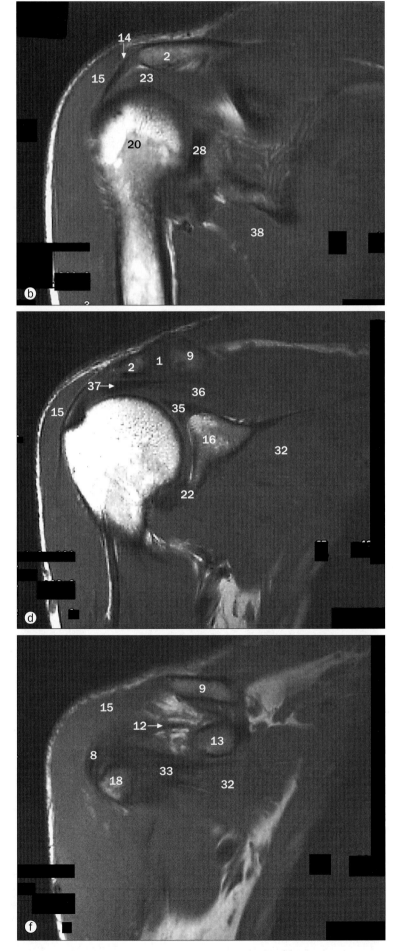

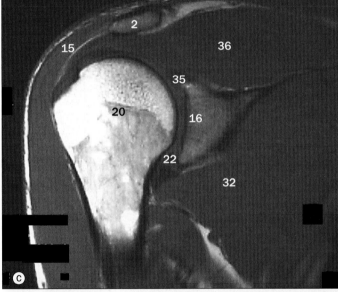

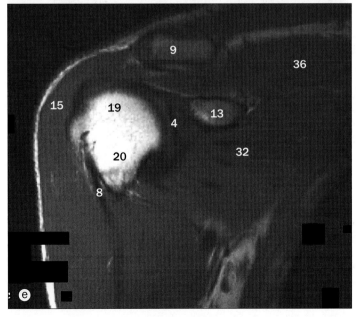

(a)–(f) Shoulder, coronal oblique MR images. See pages 74 and 75 for key.

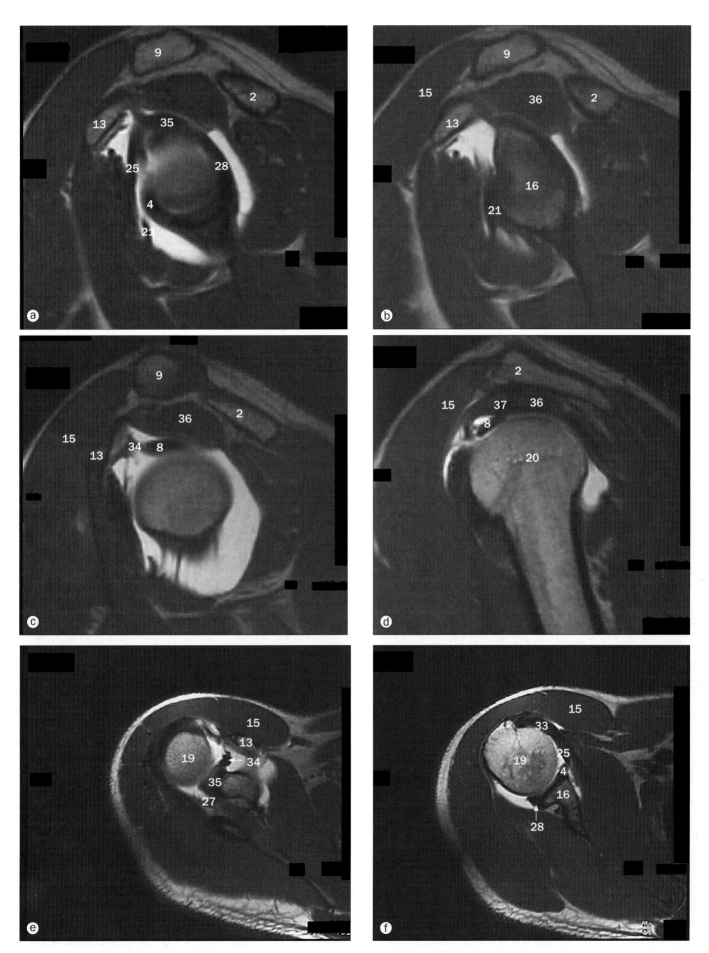

Post gadolinium arthrogram, MR images. (a)–(d) Sagittal oblique projection, (e)–(h) axial projection, (i)–(l) coronal oblique projection. See pages 74 and 75 for key.

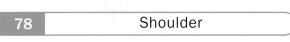

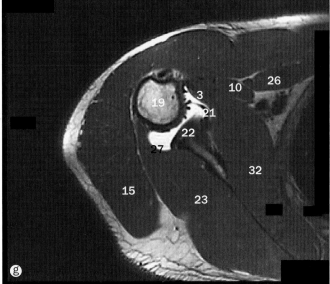

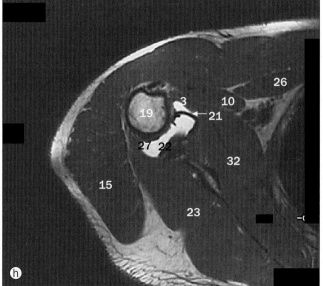

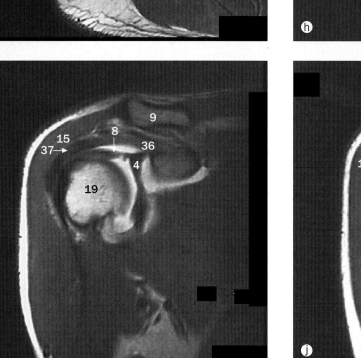

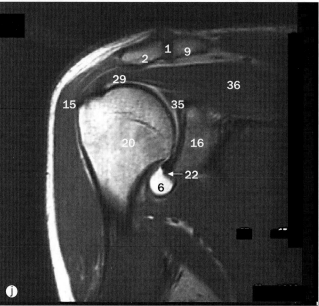

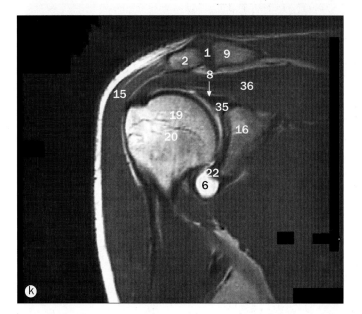

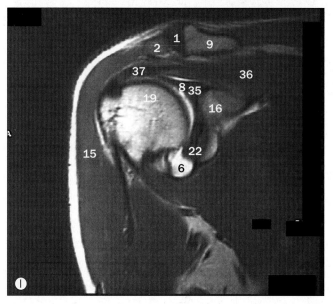

Post gadolinium arthrogram, MR images. (g) and (h) axial projection, (i)–(l) coronal oblique projection.
See pages 74 and 75 for key.

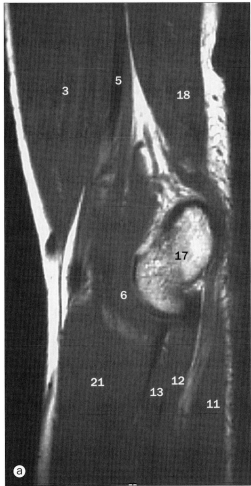

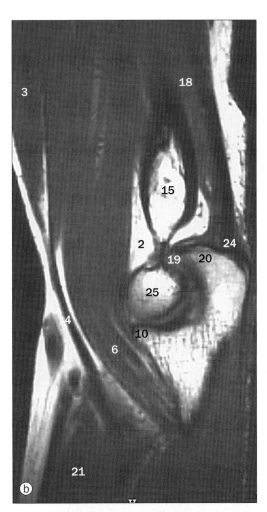

(a)–(d) Elbow, sagittal MR images.

1 Abductor pollicis longus muscle
2 Anterior fat pad
3 Biceps brachii muscle
4 Biceps brachii tendon
5 Brachial artery
6 Brachialis muscle
7 Brachioradialis muscle
8 Capitulum of humerus
9 Cephalic vein
10 Coronoid process of ulna
11 Flexor carpi ulnaris muscle
12 Flexor digitorum profundus muscle
13 Flexor digitorum superficialis muscle
14 Head of radius
15 Humerus
16 Lateral head of triceps muscle
17 Medial epicondyle
18 Medial head of triceps muscle
19 Olecranon fossa of humerus
20 Olecranon process of ulna
21 Pronator teres muscle
22 Radius
23 Supinator muscle
24 Tendon of triceps muscle
25 Trochlea of humerus

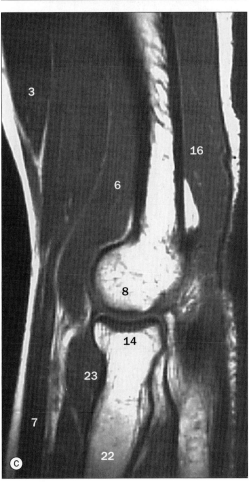

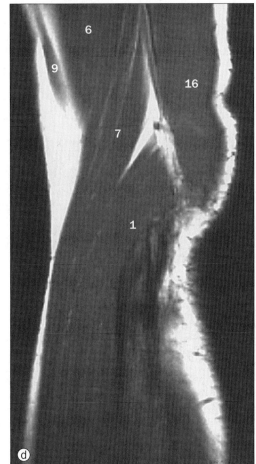

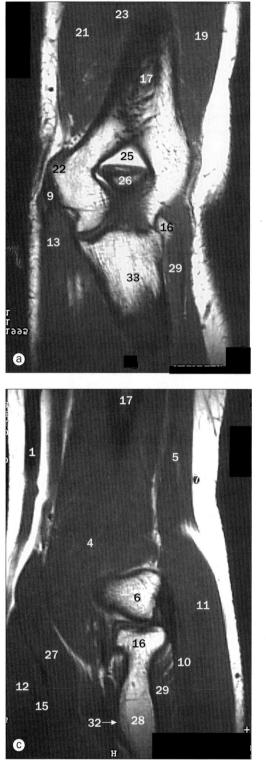

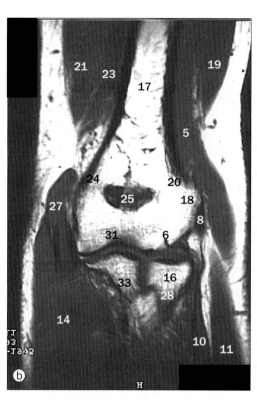

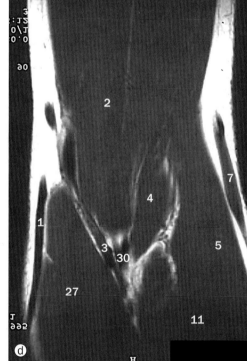

(a)–(d) Elbow, coronal MR images.

1 Basilic vein
2 Biceps brachii muscle
3 Brachial artery
4 Brachialis muscle
5 Brachioradialis muscle
6 Capitulum of humerus
7 Cephalic vein
8 Common extensor origin
9 Common flexor origin
10 Extensor carpi radialis brevis muscle
11 Extensor carpi radialis longus muscle
12 Flexor carpi radialis muscle
13 Flexor carpi ulnaris muscle
14 Flexor digitorum profundus muscle
15 Flexor digitorum superficialis muscle
16 Head of radius
17 Humerus
18 Lateral epicondyle
19 Lateral head of triceps muscle
20 Lateral supracondylar ridge
21 Long head of triceps muscle
22 Medial epicondyle
23 Medial head of triceps muscle
24 Medial supracondylar ridge
25 Olecranon fossa of humerus
26 Olecranon process of ulna
27 Pronator teres muscle
28 Radius
29 Supinator muscle
30 Tendon of biceps brachii muscle
31 Trochlea of humerus
32 Tuberosity of radius
33 Ulna

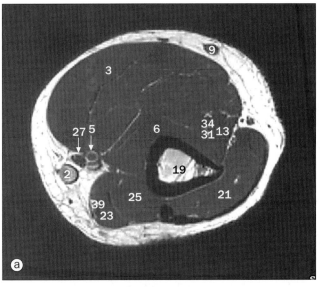

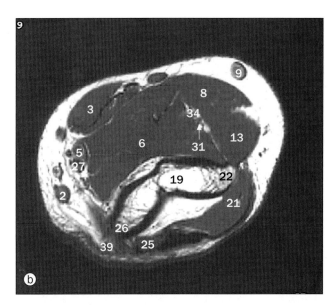

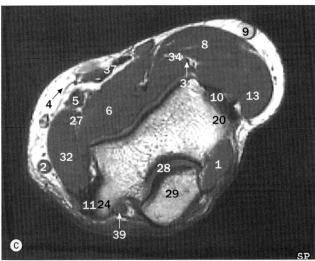

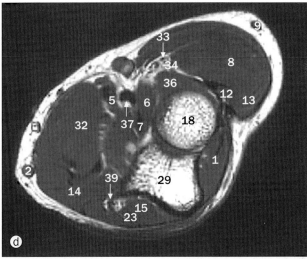

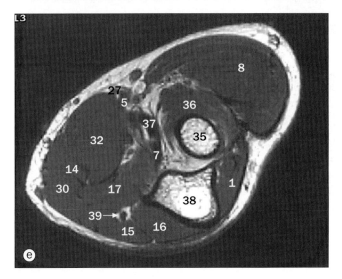

(a)–(e) Elbow, axial MR images.

1 Anconeus muscle	20 Lateral epicondyle
2 Basilic vein	21 Lateral head of triceps muscle
3 Biceps brachii muscle	22 Lateral supracondylar ridge
4 Bicipital aponeurosis	23 Long head of triceps muscle
5 Brachial artery	24 Medial epicondyle
6 Brachialis muscle	25 Medial head of triceps muscle
7 Brachialis tendon	26 Medial supracondylar ridge
8 Brachioradialis muscle	27 Median nerve
9 Cephalic vein	28 Olecranon fossa of humerus
10 Common extensor origin	29 Olecranon process of ulna
11 Common flexor origin	30 Palmaris longus muscle
12 Extensor carpi radialis brevis muscle	31 Profunda brachii artery
13 Extensor carpi radialis longus muscle	32 Pronator teres muscle
14 Flexor carpi radialis muscle	33 Radial artery
15 Flexor carpi ulnaris muscle	34 Radial nerve
16 Flexor digitorum profundus muscle	35 Radius
17 Flexor digitorum superficialis muscle	36 Supinator muscle
18 Head of radius	37 Tendon of biceps brachii muscle
19 Humerus	38 Ulna
	39 Ulnar nerve

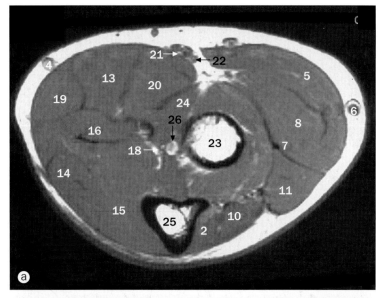

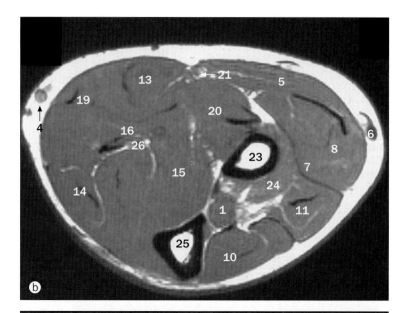

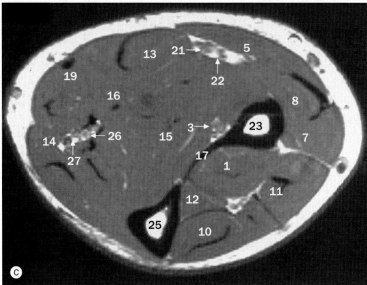

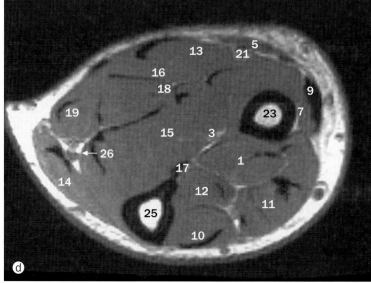

(a)–(d) Forearm, axial MR images.

1 Abductor pollicis longus muscle	**15** Flexor digitorum profundus muscle
2 Anconeus muscle	**16** Flexor digitorum superficialis muscle
3 Anterior interosseous artery	**17** Interosseous membrane
4 Basilic vein	**18** Median nerve
5 Brachioradialis muscle	**19** Palmaris longus muscle
6 Cephalic vein	**20** Pronator teres muscle
7 Extensor carpi radialis brevis muscle	**21** Radial artery
8 Extensor carpi radialis longus muscle	**22** Radial nerve
9 Extensor carpi radialis longus tendon	**23** Radius
10 Extensor carpi ulnaris muscle	**24** Supinator muscle
11 Extensor digitorum muscle	**25** Ulna
12 Extensor pollicis longus muscle	**26** Ulnar artery
13 Flexor carpi radialis muscle	**27** Ulnar nerve
14 Flexor carpi ulnaris muscle	

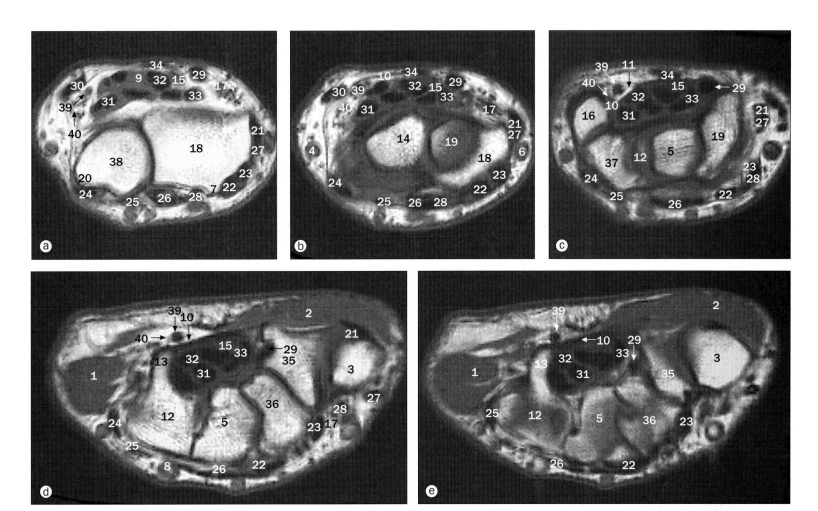

(a)–(e) Wrist, axial MR images.

1	Abductor digiti minimi muscle	**21**	Tendon of abductor pollicis longus muscle
2	Abductor pollicis brevis muscle	**22**	Tendon of extensor carpi radialis brevis muscle
3	Base of first metacarpal	**23**	Tendon of extensor carpi radialis longus muscle
4	Basilic vein	**24**	Tendon of extensor carpi ulnaris muscle
5	Capitate	**25**	Tendon of extensor digiti minimi muscle
6	Cephalic vein	**26**	Tendon of extensor digitorum muscle
7	Dorsal tubercle of radius	**27**	Tendon of extensor pollicis brevis muscle
8	Dorsal venous arch	**28**	Tendon of extensor pollicis longus muscle
9	Flexor digitorum superficialis muscle	**29**	Tendon of flexor carpi radialis muscle
10	Flexor retinaculum	**30**	Tendon of flexor carpi ulnaris muscle
11	Guyon's canal	**31**	Tendon of flexor digitorum profundus muscle
12	Hamate	**32**	Tendon of flexor digitorum superficialis muscle
13	Hook of hamate	**33**	Tendon of flexor pollicis longus muscle
14	Lunate	**34**	Tendon of palmaris longus muscle
15	Median nerve	**35**	Trapezium
16	Pisiform	**36**	Trapezoid
17	Radial artery	**37**	Triquetral
18	Radius	**38**	Ulna
19	Scaphoid	**39**	Ulnar artery
20	Styloid process of ulna	**40**	Ulnar nerve

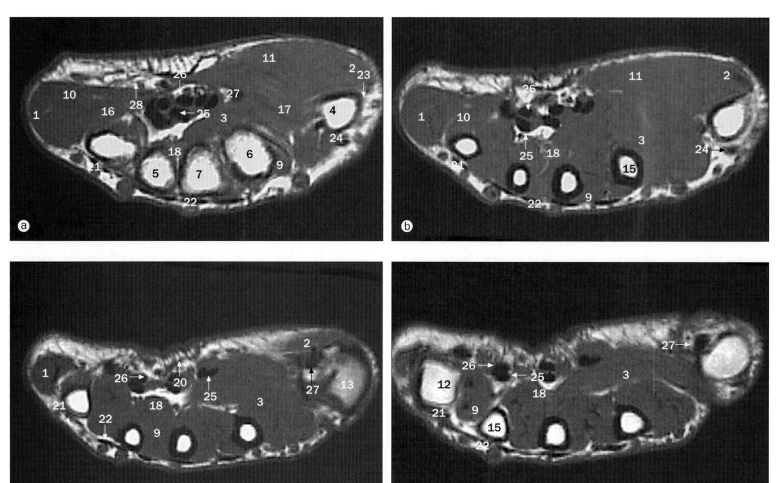

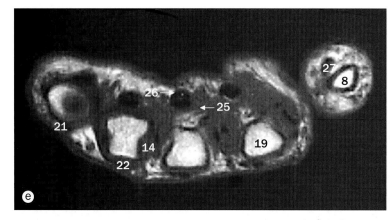

(a)–(e) Hand, axial MR images.

1	Abductor digiti minimi muscle	**19**	Proximal phalanx of index finger
2	Abductor pollicis brevis muscle	**20**	Superficial palmar arch
3	Adductor pollicis muscle	**21**	Tendon of extensor digiti minimi muscle
4	Base of first metacarpal		
5	Base of fourth metacarpal	**22**	Tendon of extensor digitorum muscle
6	Base of second metacarpal		
7	Base of third metacarpal	**23**	Tendon of extensor pollicis brevis muscle
8	Distal phalanx of thumb		
9	Dorsal interossei muscles	**24**	Tendon of extensor pollicis longus muscle
10	Flexor digiti minimi muscle		
11	Flexor pollicis brevis muscle	**25**	Tendon of flexor digitorum profundus muscle
12	Head of fifth metacarpal		
13	Head of first metacarpal	**26**	Tendon of flexor digitorum superficialis muscle
14	Lumbrical muscle		
15	Metacarpal shaft	**27**	Tendon of flexor pollicis longus muscle
16	Opponens digiti minimi muscle		
17	Opponens pollicis muscle	**28**	Ulnar artery
18	Palmar interossei muscles		

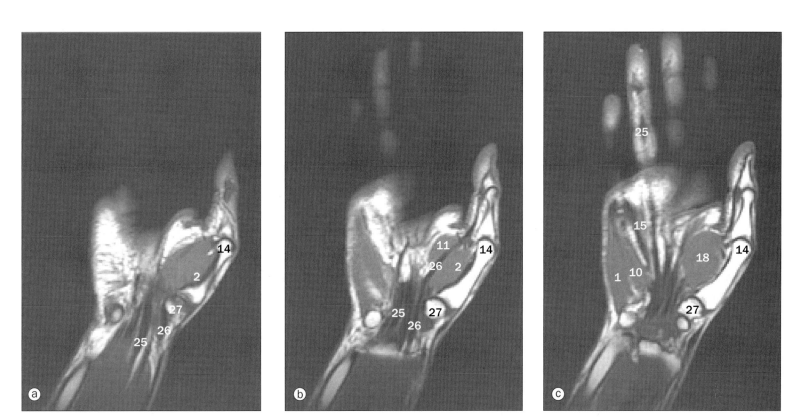

(a)–(h) Hand, coronal MR images.

1 Abductor digiti minimi muscle	**15** Lumbrical muscle
2 Abductor pollicis brevis muscle	**16** Middle phalanx
3 Adductor pollicis muscle	**17** Opponens digiti minimi muscle
4 Base of proximal phalanx	**18** Opponens pollicis muscle
5 Capitate	**19** Palmar interossei muscles
6 Common palmar digital artery	**20** Proper palmar digital artery
7 Deep palmar arch	**21** Proximal phalanx of thumb
8 Distal phalanx of thumb	**22** Shaft of proximal phalanx
9 Dorsal interossei muscles	**23** Tendon of extensor pollicis longus muscle
10 Flexor digiti minimi muscle	**24** Tendon of flexor digitorum profundus muscle
11 Flexor pollicis brevis muscle	**25** Tendon of flexor digitorum superficialis muscle
12 Hamate	**26** Tendon of flexor pollicis longus muscle
13 Head of fifth metacarpal	**27** Trapezium
14 Head of first metacarpal	**28** Trapezoid

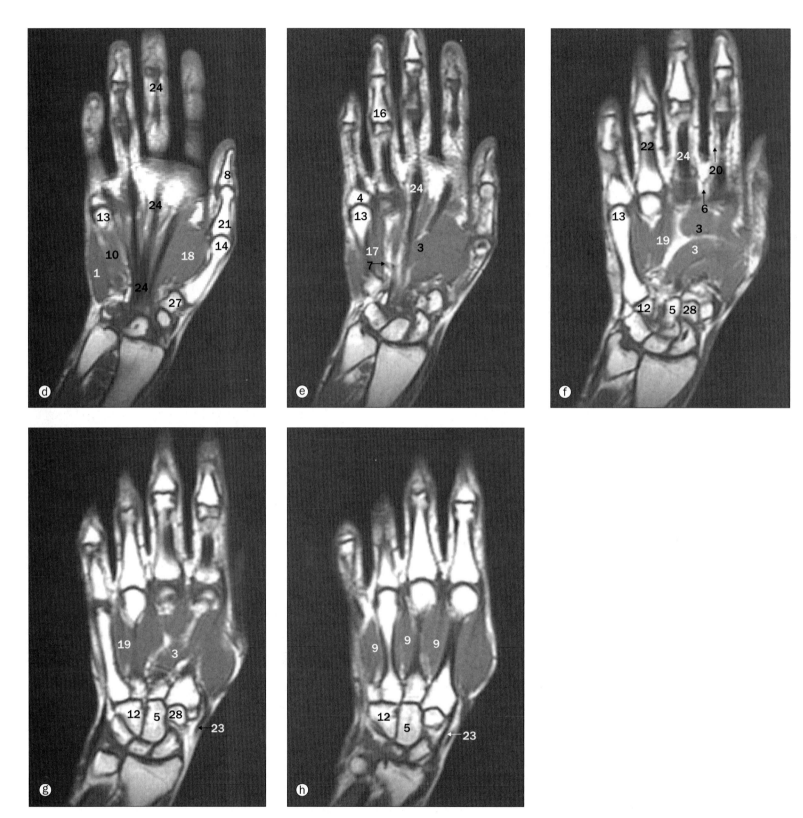

(d)–(h) Hand, coronal MR images. See page 85 for key.

4 Thorax

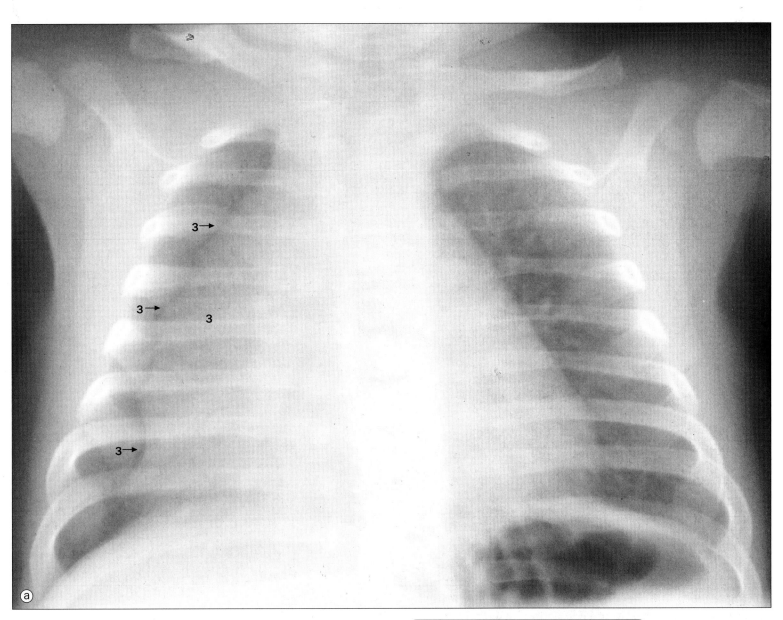

(a) Chest of a 4-month-old child, postero-anterior radiograph.
(b) Cervical rib, adult, postero-anterior projection.
(c) Azygos fissure, adult, postero-anterior projection.

1 Azygos fissure
2 Cervical rib
3 Thymus

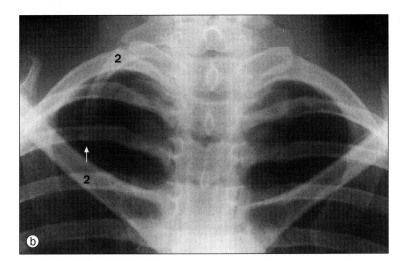

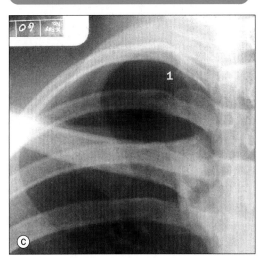

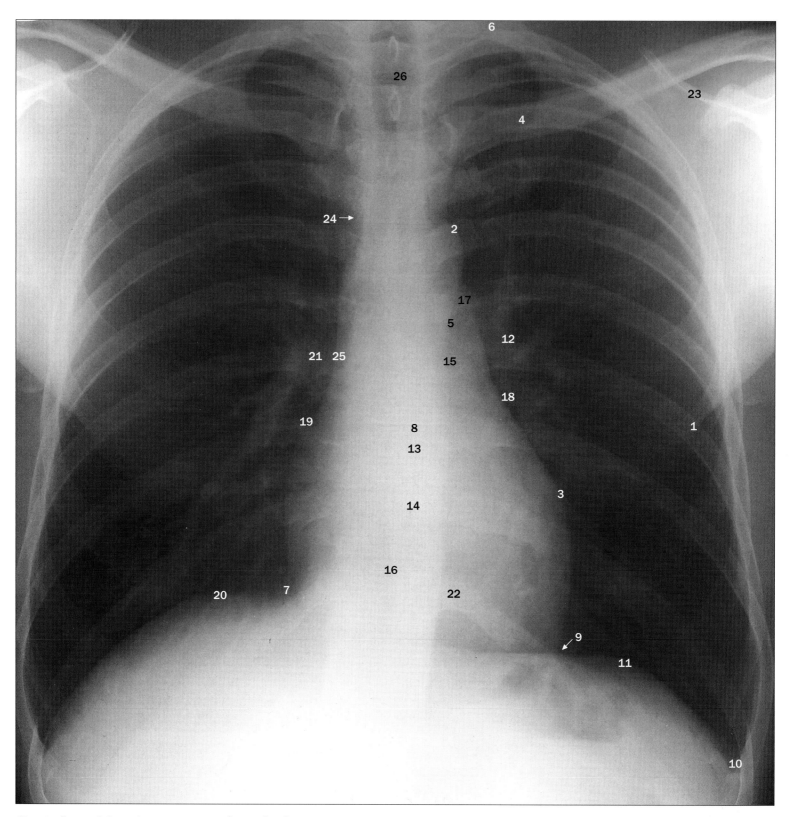

Chest of an adult male, postero-anterior projection.

1 Anterior axillary fold	**10** Left costophrenic angle	**19** Right atrial border
2 Arch of aorta (aortic knuckle or knob)	**11** Left dome of diaphragm	**20** Right dome of diaphragm
3 Border of left ventricle	**12** Left pulmonary artery	**21** Right pulmonary artery
4 Clavicle	**13** Position of aortic valve	**22** Right ventricle
5 Descending aorta	**14** Position of mitral valve	**23** Spine of scapula
6 First rib	**15** Position of pulmonary valve	**24** Sternum
7 Inferior vena cava	**16** Position of tricuspid valve	**25** Superior vena cava
8 Left atrium	**17** Pulmonary trunk	**26** Trachea
9 Left cardiophrenic angle	**18** Region of tip of auricle of left atrium	

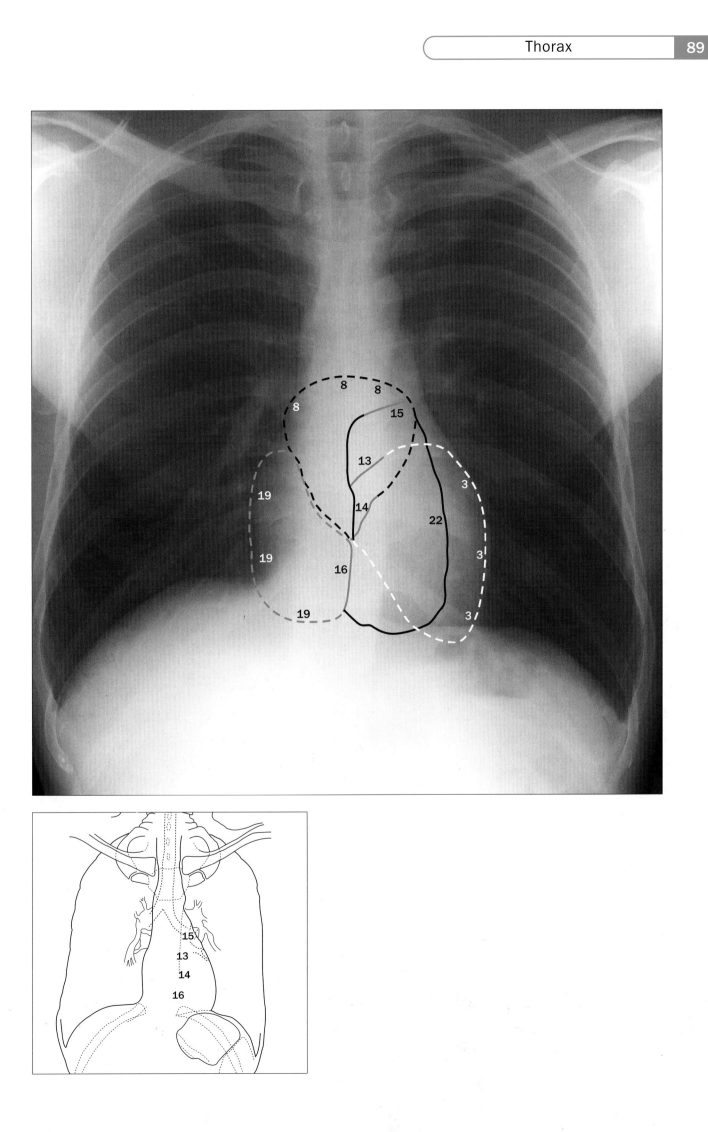

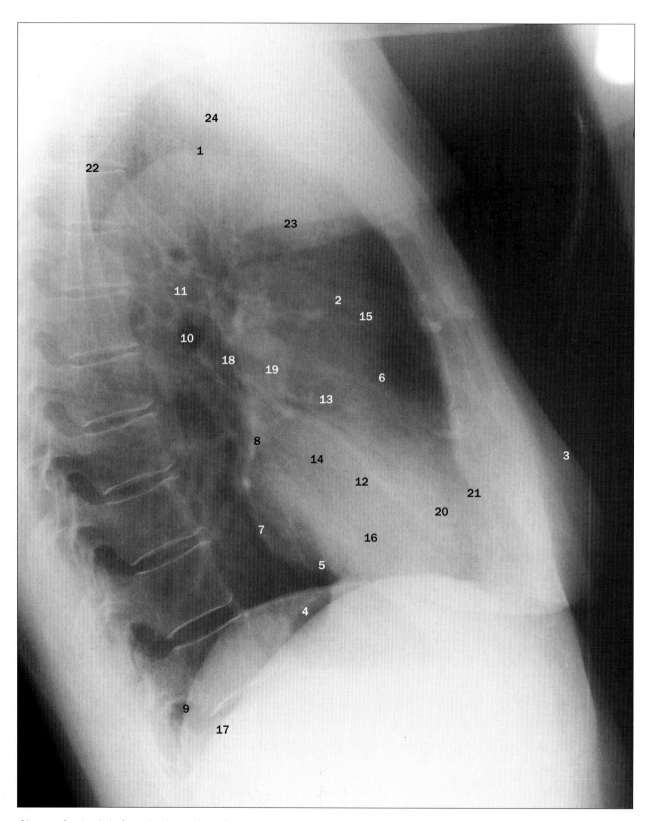

Chest of an adult female, lateral projection.

1 Arch of aorta (aortic knuckle or knob)	**9** Left dome of diaphragm	**18** Right main bronchus
2 Ascending aorta	**10** Left main bronchus	**19** Right main pulmonary artery
3 Breast	**11** Left main pulmonary artery	**20** Right ventricle
4 Gas in fundus of stomach	**12** Left oblique fissure	**21** Right ventricular border of heart
5 Inferior vena cava	**13** Position of aortic valve	**22** Scapula
6 Infundibulum of right ventricle (below)	**14** Position of mitral valve	**23** Soft tissues of upper arm
with pulmonary trunk (above)	**15** Position of pulmonary valve	**24** Trachea
7 Left atrial border of heart	**16** Position of tricuspid valve	
8 Left atrium	**17** Right dome of diaphragm	

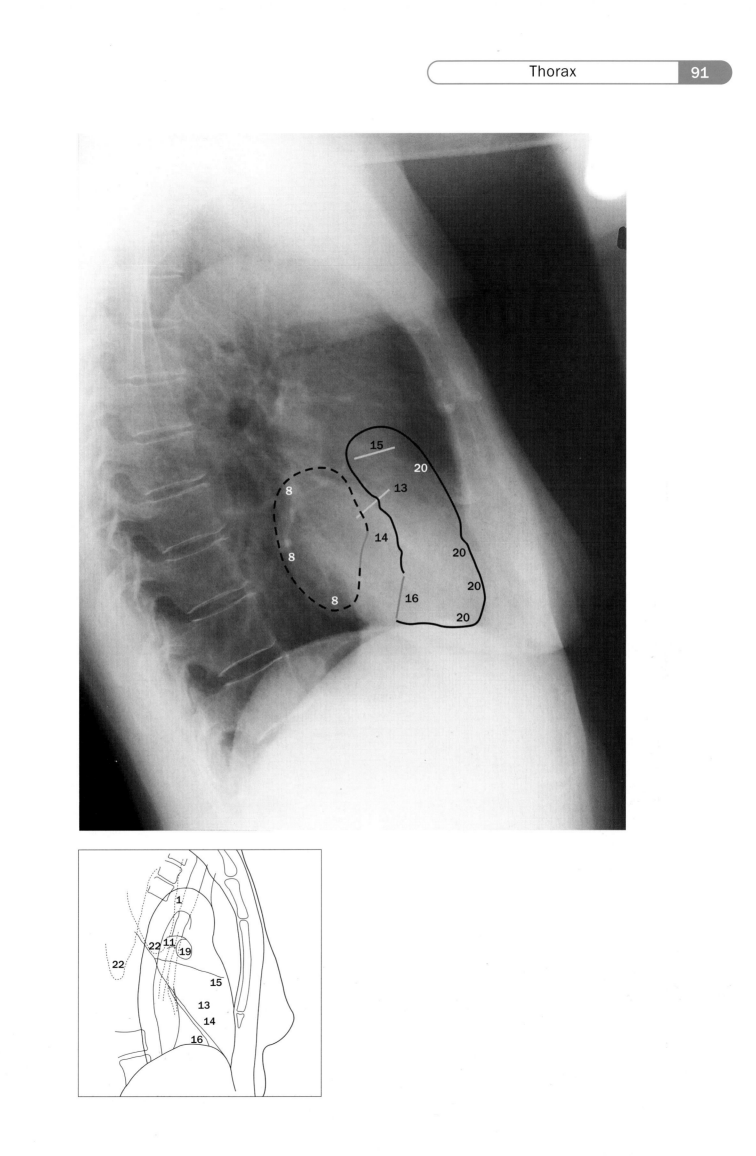

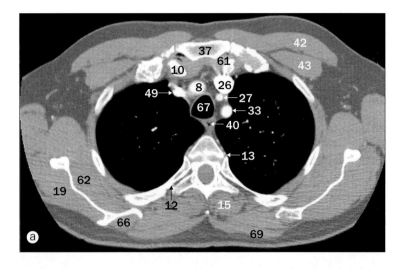

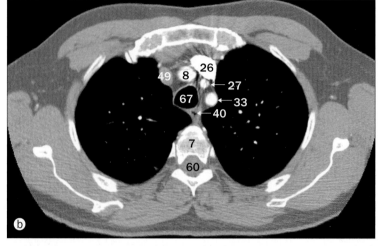

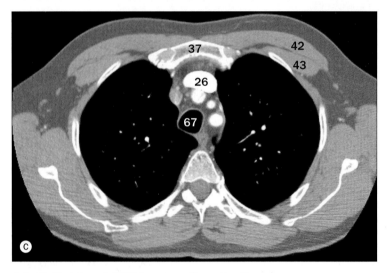

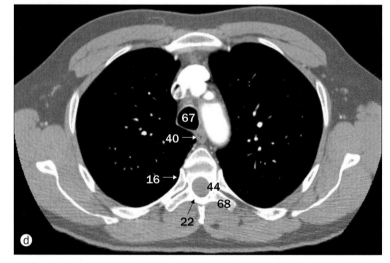

(a)–(t) Chest, axial CT images of mediastinum.

1	Anterior interventricular branch of left coronary artery	**19**	Infraspinatus muscle
2	Aortic valve	**20**	Interatrial septum
3	Arch of aorta (aortic knuckle or knob)	**21**	Internal thoracic artery and vein
4	Ascending aorta	**22**	Lamina
5	Azygos vein	**23**	Latissimus dorsi muscle
6	Body of sternum	**24**	Left atrial appendage (auricle)
7	Body of vertebra	**25**	Left atrium
8	Brachiocephalic trunk	**26**	Left brachiocephalic vein
9	Carina (bifurcation of trachea)	**27**	Left common carotid artery
10	Clavicle	**28**	Left hemidiaphragm
11	Coronary sinus	**29**	Left inferior lobe bronchus
12	Costotransverse joint	**30**	Left inferior pulmonary vein
13	Costovertebral joint	**31**	Left main bronchus
14	Descending aorta	**32**	Left pulmonary artery
15	Erector spinae muscle	**33**	Left subclavian artery
16	Head of rib	**34**	Left superior lobe bronchus
17	Hemi-azygos vein	**35**	Left superior pulmonary vein
18	Inferior vena cava	**36**	Left ventricular cavity

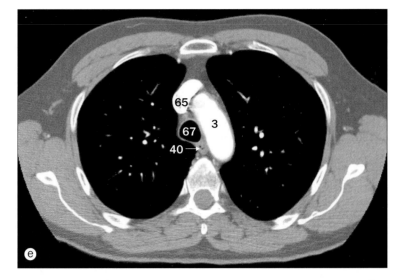

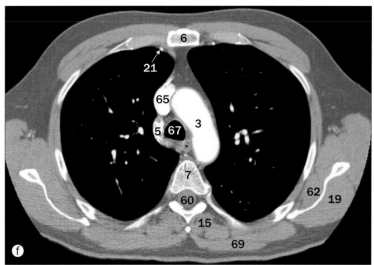

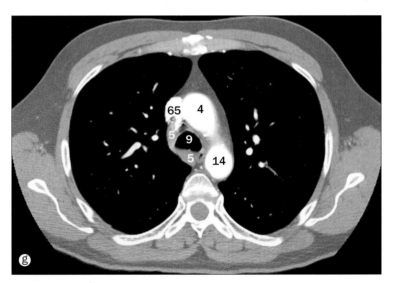

(e)–(h) Chest, axial CT images of mediastinum.

37 Manubrium of sternum	**55** Right pulmonary artery
38 Mitral valve	**56** Right superior lobe bronchus
39 Muscular interventricular septum	**57** Right superior pulmonary vein
40 Oesophagus	**58** Right ventricular cavity
41 Papillary muscles	**59** Serratus anterior muscle
42 Pectoralis major muscle	**60** Spinal canal
43 Pectoralis minor muscle	**61** Sternoclavicular joint
44 Pedicle	**62** Subscapularis muscle
45 Pericardium	**63** Superior lobe branch of right pulmonary artery
46 Pulmonary trunk	**64** Superior pericardial recess
47 Right atrial appendage (auricle)	**65** Superior vena cava
48 Right atrium	**66** Supraspinatus muscle
49 Right brachiocephalic vein	**67** Trachea
50 Right hemidiaphragm	**68** Transverse process
51 Right inferior lobe bronchus	**69** Trapezius muscle
52 Right inferior pulmonary vein	**70** Tricuspid valve
53 Right lobe of liver	**71** Xiphisternum
54 Right main bronchus	

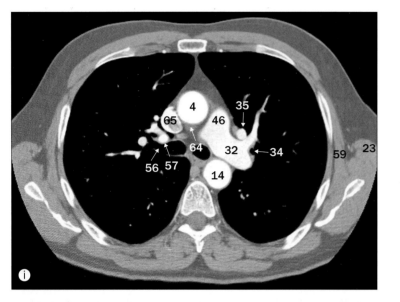

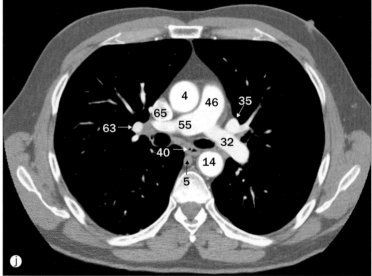

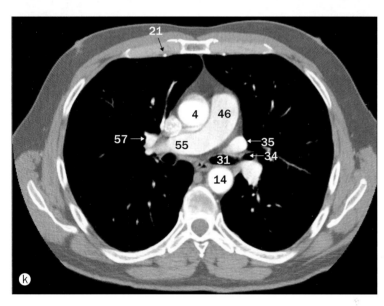

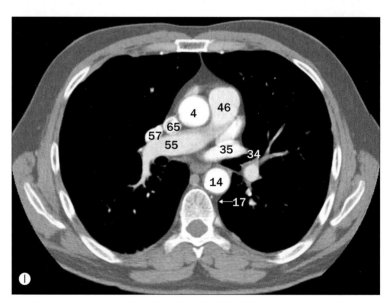

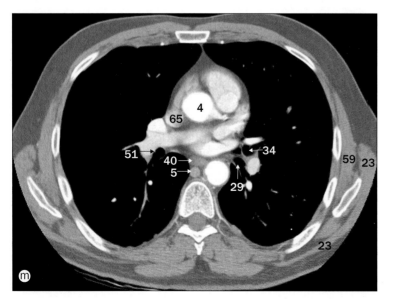

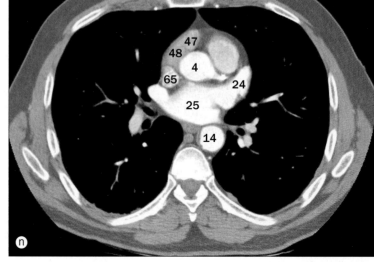

(i)–(n) Chest, axial CT images of mediastinum. See pages 92–93 for key.

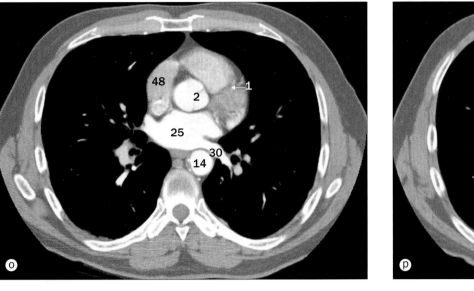

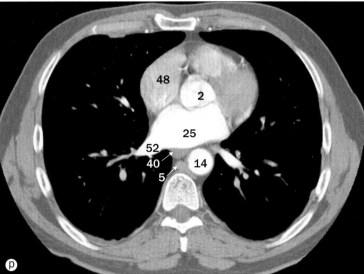

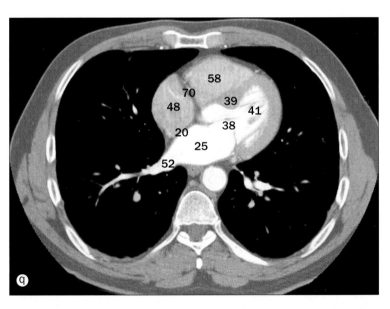

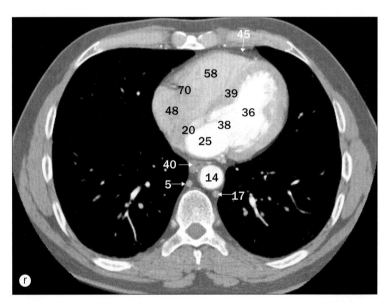

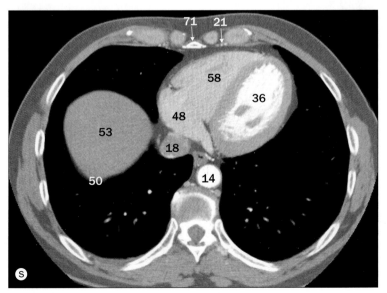

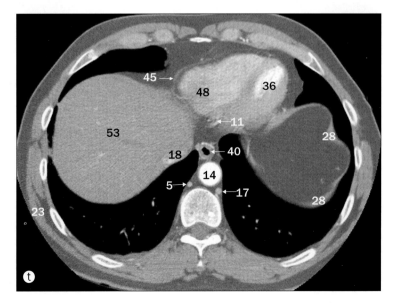

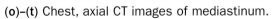

(o)–(t) Chest, axial CT images of mediastinum.

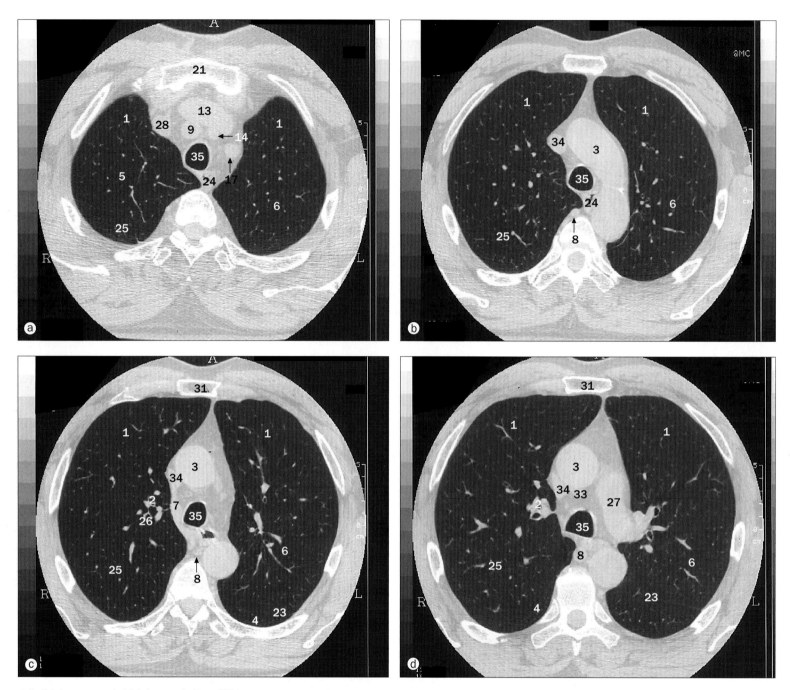

(a)–(h) Lungs, axial high resolution CT images.

1 Anterior segment superior lobe	**11** Horizontal fissure
2 Anterior segmental bronchus	**12** Lateral segment middle lobe
3 Aorta	**13** Left brachiocephalic vein
4 Apical segment inferior lobe	**14** Left common carotid artery
5 Apical segment right superior lobe	**15** Left inferior lobe bronchus
6 Apicoposterior segment left superior lobe	**16** Left main bronchus
7 Azygos arch	**17** Left subclavian artery
8 Azygos vein	**18** Left superior lobe bronchus
9 Brachiocephalic trunk	**19** Left superior pulmonary vein
10 Bronchus intermedius	**20** Lingular segmental bronchus

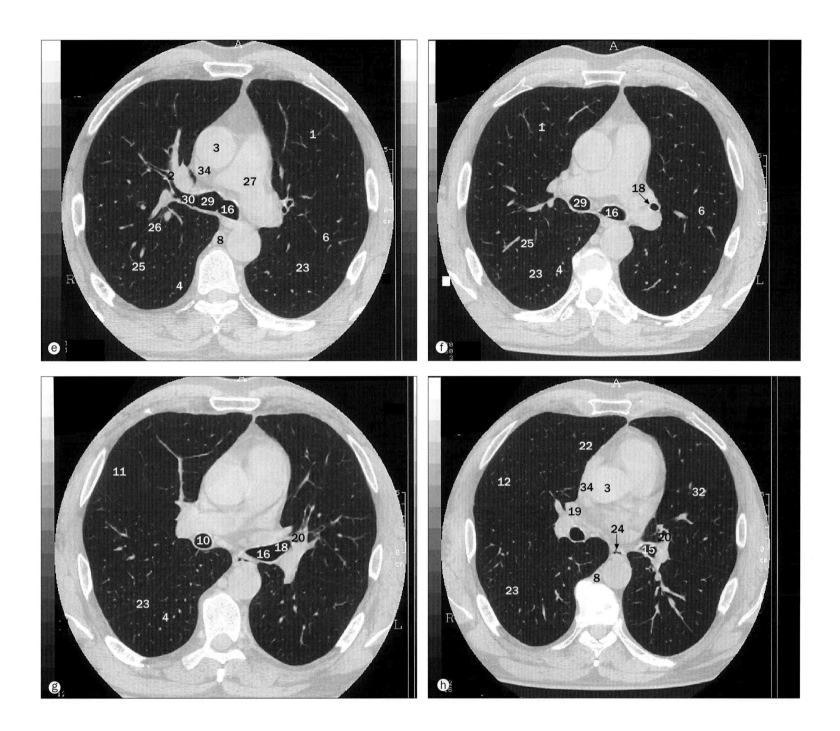

21 Manubrium of sternum
22 Medial segment middle lobe
23 Oblique fissure
24 Oesophagus
25 Posterior segment superior lobe
26 Posterior segmental bronchus
27 Pulmonary artery
28 Right brachiocephalic vein

29 Right main bronchus
30 Right superior lobe bronchus
31 Sternum
32 Superior lingular segment
33 Superior pericardial recess
34 Superior vena cava
35 Trachea

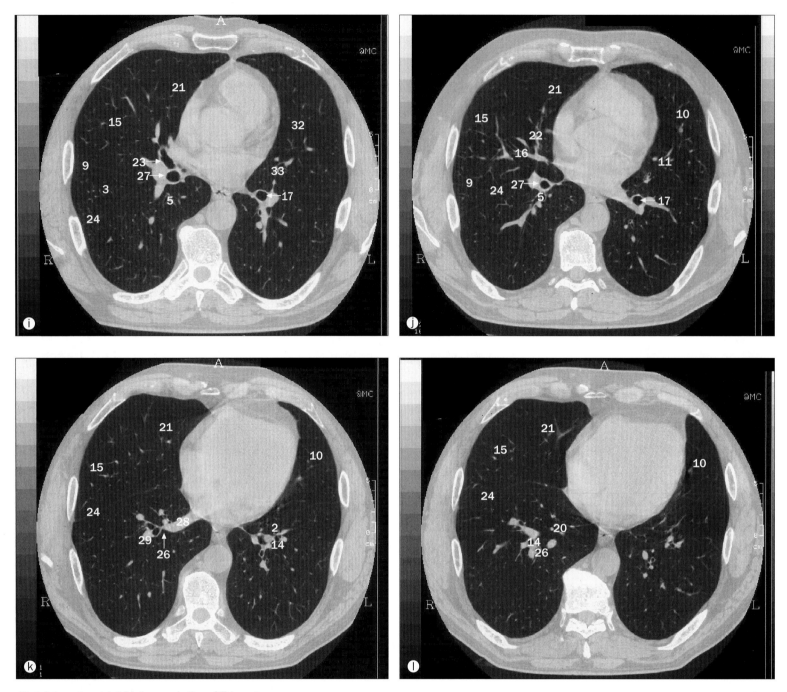

(i)–(p) Lungs, axial high resolution CT images.

1 Anterior basal segment inferior lobe	**10** Inferior lingular segment
2 Anterior basal segmental bronchus	**11** Inferior lingular segmental bronchus
3 Anterior segment superior lobe	**12** Inferior vena cava
4 Aorta	**13** Lateral basal segment inferior lobe
5 Apical segment inferior lobe bronchus	**14** Lateral basal segmental bronchus
6 Azygos vein	**15** Lateral segment middle lobe
7 Heart	**16** Lateral segmental bronchus of middle lobe
8 Hemi-azygos vein	**17** Left inferior lobe bronchus
9 Horizontal fissure	

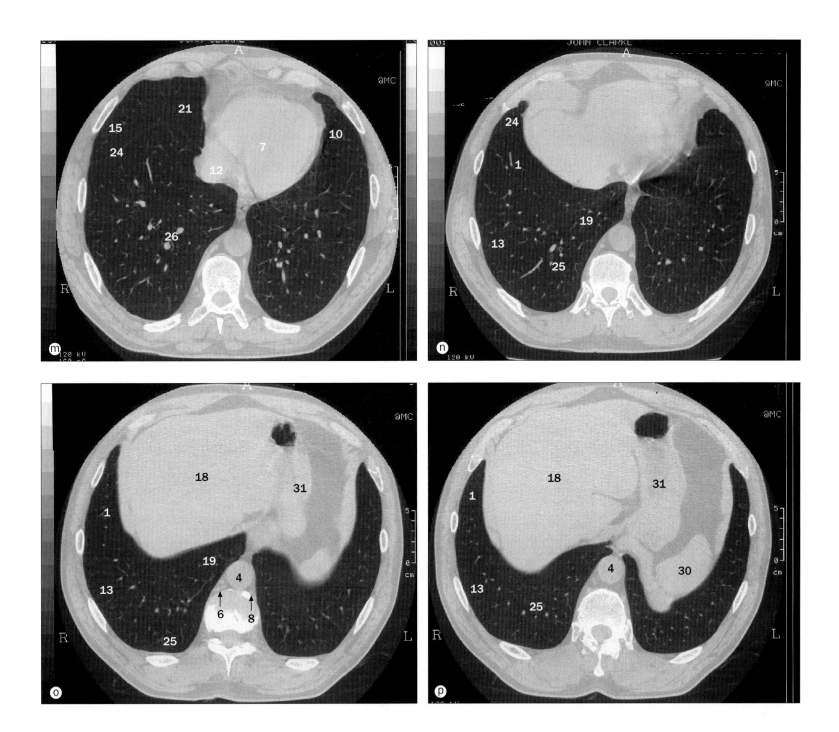

18 Liver
19 Medial basal segment inferior lobe
20 Medial basal segmental bronchus
21 Medial segment middle lobe
22 Medial segmental bronchus of middle lobe
23 Middle lobe bronchus
24 Oblique fissure
25 Posterior basal segment inferior lobe

26 Posterior basal segmental bronchus
27 Right inferior lobe bronchus
28 Right inferior pulmonary vein
29 Right lower lobe pulmonary artery
30 Spleen
31 Stomach
32 Superior lingular segment
33 Superior lingular segmental bronchus

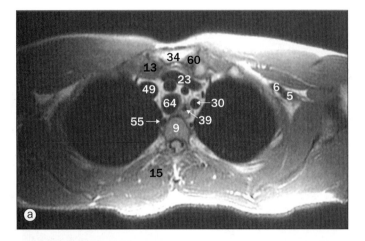

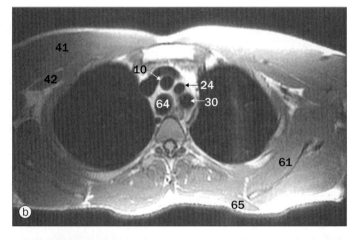

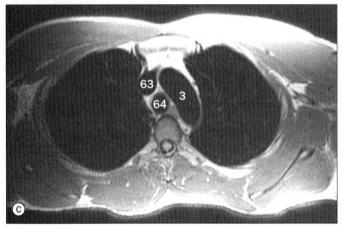

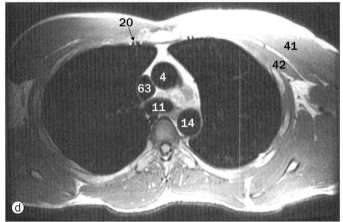

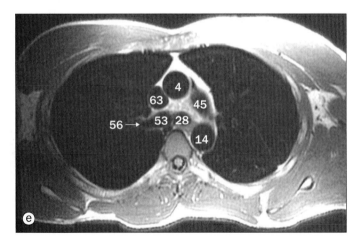

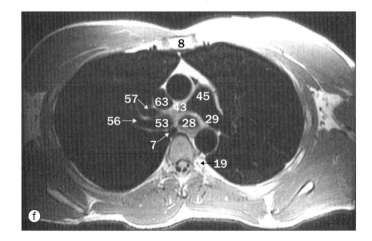

(a)–(x) Chest, axial MR images.

1 Anterior interventricular branch of left coronary artery	**12** Circumflex branch of left coronary artery	**24** Left common carotid artery
2 Aortic valve	**13** Clavicle	**25** Left coronary artery
3 Arch of aorta (aortic knuckle or knob)	**14** Descending aorta	**26** Left inferior lobe bronchus
4 Ascending aorta	**15** Erector spinae muscle	**27** Left inferior pulmonary vein
5 Axillary artery	**16** Hemi-azygos vein	**28** Left main bronchus
6 Axillary vein	**17** Inferior vena cava	**29** Left pulmonary artery
7 Azygos vein	**18** Interatrial septum	**30** Left subclavian artery
8 Body of sternum	**19** Intercostal artery	**31** Left superior lobe bronchus
9 Body of vertebra	**20** Internal thoracic artery and vein	**32** Left superior pulmonary vein
10 Brachiocephalic trunk	**21** Left atrial appendage (auricle)	**33** Left ventricular cavity
11 Carina (bifurcation of trachea)	**22** Left atrium	**34** Manubrium of sternum
	23 Left brachiocephalic vein	**35** Membranous interventricular septum

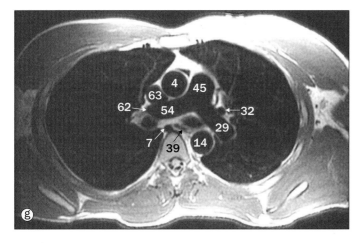

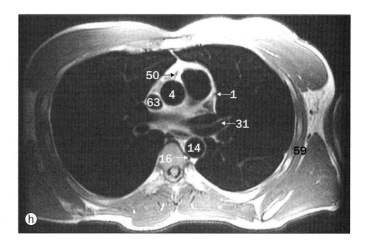

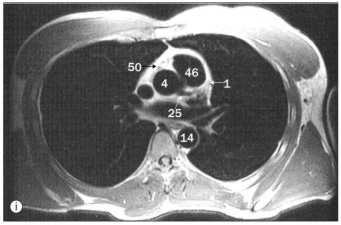

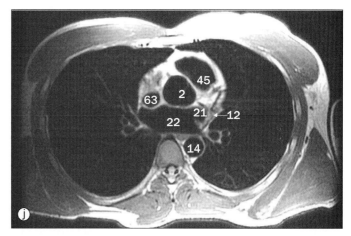

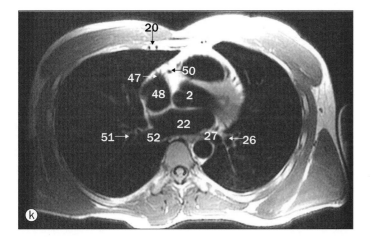

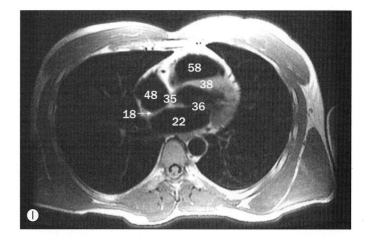

36 Mitral valve	**47** Right atrial appendage (auricle)	**58** Right ventricular cavity
37 Moderator band	**48** Right atrium	**59** Serratus anterior muscle
38 Muscular interventricular septum	**49** Right brachiocephalic vein	**60** Sternoclavicular joint
39 Oesophagus	**50** Right coronary artery	**61** Subscapularis muscle
40 Papillary muscles	**51** Right inferior lobe bronchus	**62** Superior lobe branch of
41 Pectoralis major muscle	**52** Right inferior pulmonary vein	right pulmonary artery
42 Pectoralis minor muscle	**53** Right main bronchus	**63** Superior vena cava
43 Pericardial recess	**54** Right pulmonary artery	**64** Trachea
44 Pericardium	**55** Right superior intercostal vein	**65** Trapezius muscle
45 Pulmonary trunk	**56** Right superior lobe bronchus	**66** Tricuspid valve
46 Pulmonary valve	**57** Right superior pulmonary vein	

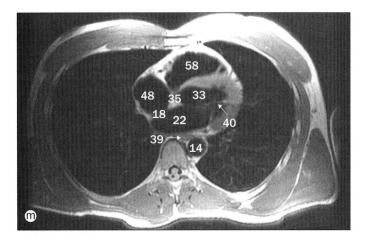

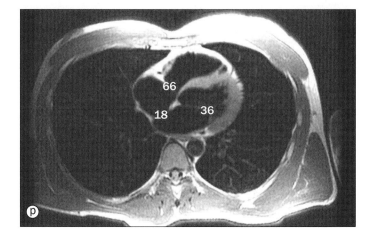

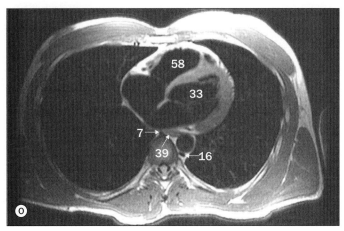

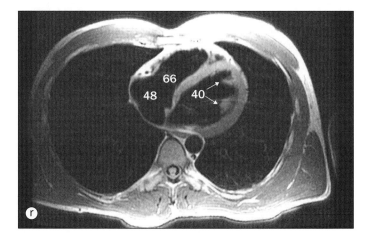

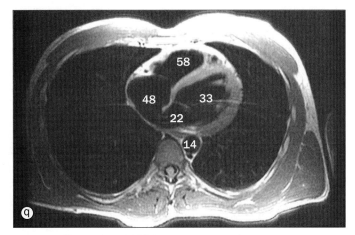

(m)–(x) Chest, axial MR images.

1 Anterior interventricular branch of left coronary artery	**12** Circumflex branch of left coronary artery	**24** Left common carotid artery
2 Aortic valve	**13** Clavicle	**25** Left coronary artery
3 Arch of aorta (aortic knuckle or knob)	**14** Descending aorta	**26** Left inferior lobe bronchus
4 Ascending aorta	**15** Erector spinae muscle	**27** Left inferior pulmonary vein
5 Axillary artery	**16** Hemi-azygos vein	**28** Left main bronchus
6 Axillary vein	**17** Inferior vena cava	**29** Left pulmonary artery
7 Azygos vein	**18** Interatrial septum	**30** Left subclavian artery
8 Body of sternum	**19** Intercostal artery	**31** Left superior lobe bronchus
9 Body of vertebra	**20** Internal thoracic artery and vein	**32** Left superior pulmonary vein
10 Brachiocephalic trunk	**21** Left atrial appendage (auricle)	**33** Left ventricular cavity
11 Carina (bifurcation of trachea)	**22** Left atrium	**34** Manubrium of sternum
	23 Left brachiocephalic vein	**35** Membranous interventricular septum

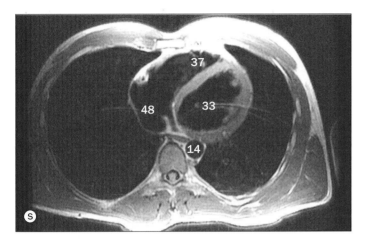

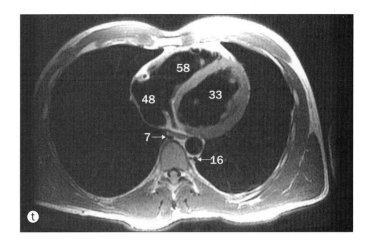

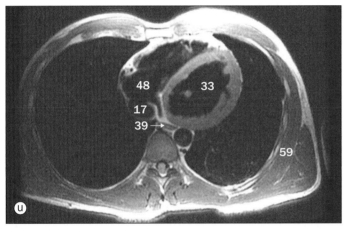

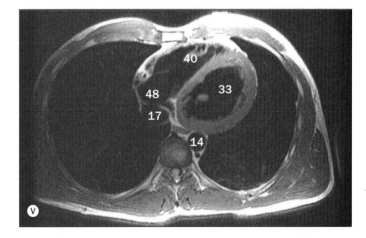

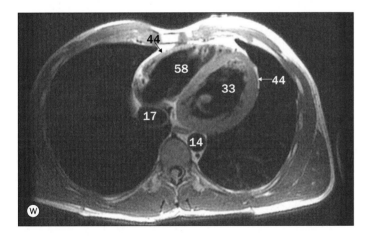

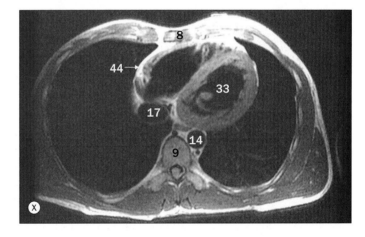

36 Mitral valve	**47** Right atrial appendage (auricle)	**58** Right ventricular cavity
37 Moderator band	**48** Right atrium	**59** Serratus anterior muscle
38 Muscular interventricular septum	**49** Right brachiocephalic vein	**60** Sternoclavicular joint
39 Oesophagus	**50** Right coronary artery	**61** Subscapularis muscle
40 Papillary muscles	**51** Right inferior lobe bronchus	**62** Superior lobe branch of
41 Pectoralis major muscle	**52** Right inferior pulmonary vein	right pulmonary artery
42 Pectoralis minor muscle	**53** Right main bronchus	**63** Superior vena cava
43 Pericardial recess	**54** Right pulmonary artery	**64** Trachea
44 Pericardium	**55** Right superior intercostal vein	**65** Trapezius muscle
45 Pulmonary trunk	**56** Right superior lobe bronchus	**66** Tricuspid valve
46 Pulmonary valve	**57** Right superior pulmonary vein	

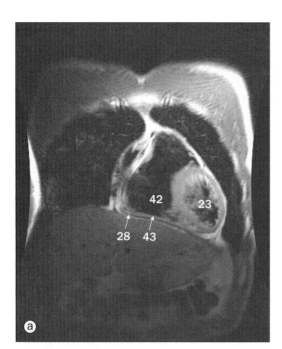

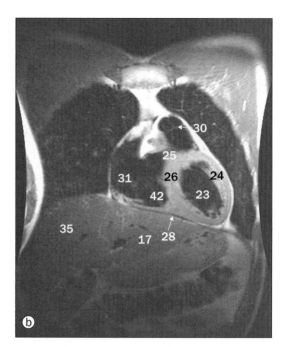

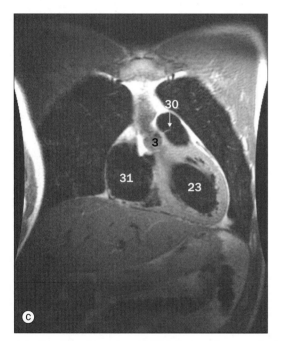

(a)–(h) Chest, coronal MR images, from anterior to posterior.

1 Aortic valve	**13** Left atrium
2 Arch of aorta (aortic knuckle or knob)	**14** Left brachiocephalic vein
3 Ascending aorta	**15** Left common carotid artery
4 Brachiocephalic trunk	**16** Left coronary artery
5 Carina (bifurcation of trachea)	**17** Left lobe of liver
6 Clavicle	**18** Left main bronchus
7 Coronary sinus	**19** Left pulmonary artery
8 Descending aorta	**20** Left subclavian artery
9 Hepatic veins	**21** Left subclavian artery
10 Inferior vena cava	**22** Left superior pulmonary vein
11 Interatrial septum	**23** Left ventricular cavity
12 Left atrial appendage (auricle)	**24** Left ventricular wall

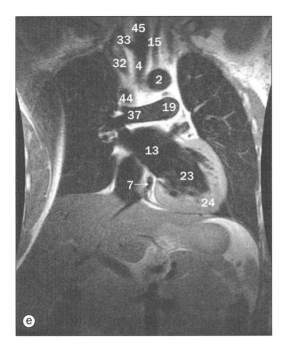

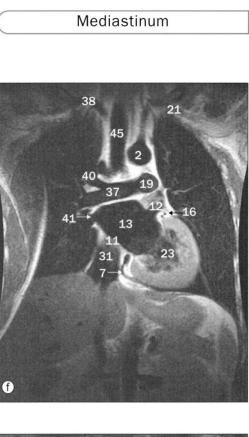

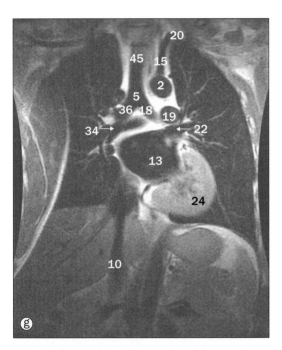

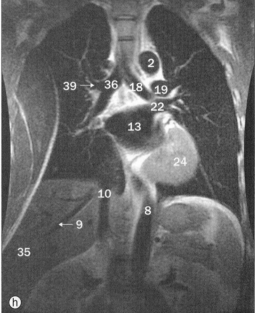

25	Membranous interventricular septum	36	Right main bronchus
26	Muscular interventricular septum	37	Right pulmonary artery
27	Papillary muscles	38	Right subclavian artery
28	Pericardium	39	Right superior lobe bronchus
29	Pulmonary trunk	40	Right superior lobe pulmonary artery
30	Pulmonary valve	41	Right superior pulmonary vein
31	Right atrium	42	Right ventricular cavity
32	Right brachiocephalic vein	43	Right ventricular wall
33	Right common carotid artery	44	Superior vena cava
34	Right inferior lobe bronchus	45	Trachea
35	Right lobe of liver		

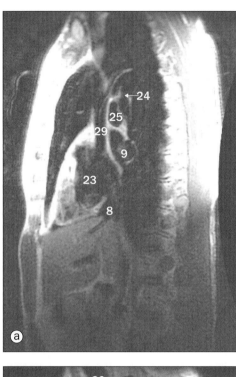

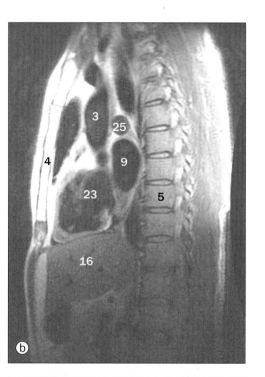

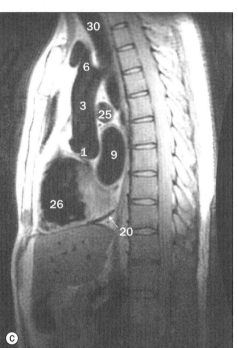

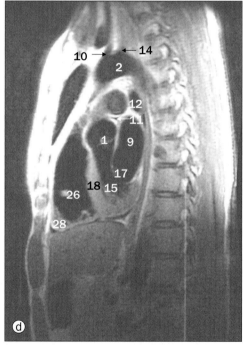

(a)–(h) Chest, sagittal MR images.

1 Aortic valve	**9** Left atrium
2 Arch of aorta (aortic knuckle or knob)	**10** Left common carotid artery
3 Ascending aorta	**11** Left coronary artery
4 Body of sternum	**12** Left main bronchus
5 Body of vertebra	**13** Left pulmonary artery
6 Brachiocephalic trunk	**14** Left subclavian artery
7 Descending aorta	**15** Left ventricular cavity
8 Inferior vena cava	**16** Liver

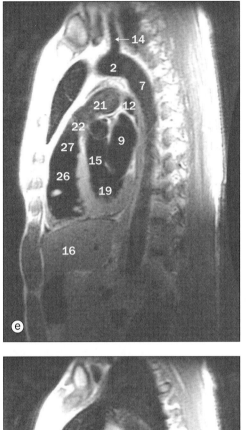

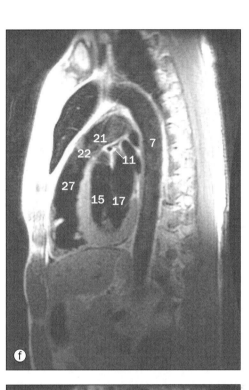

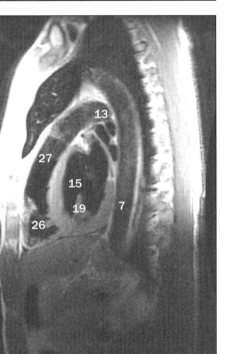

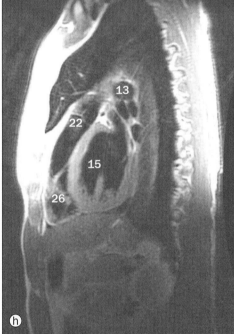

17 Mitral valve
18 Muscular interventricular septum
19 Papillary muscles
20 Pericardium
21 Pulmonary trunk
22 Pulmonary valve
23 Right atrium

24 Right main bronchus
25 Right pulmonary artery
26 Right ventricular cavity
27 Right ventricular outflow tract
28 Right ventricular wall
29 Superior vena cava
30 Trachea

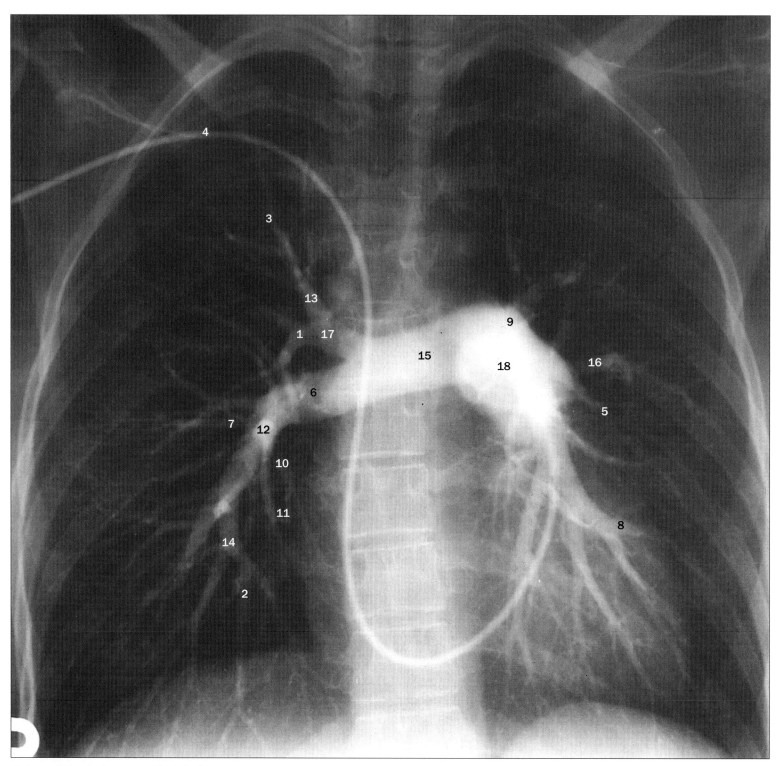

Pulmonary arteriogram, arterial phase.

1 Anterior artery (superior lobe)	**10** Medial artery (middle lobe)
2 Anterior basal artery	**11** Medial basal artery
3 Apical artery (superior lobe)	**12** Middle lobe pulmonary artery
4 Catheter introduced via right brachial vein	**13** Posterior artery (superior lobe)
5 Inferior lingular artery	**14** Posterior basal artery
6 Inferior lobe pulmonary artery	**15** Right pulmonary artery
7 Lateral artery (middle lobe)	**16** Superior lingular artery
8 Lateral basal artery	**17** Superior lobe pulmonary artery
9 Left pulmonary artery	**18** Tip of catheter in main pulmonary artery

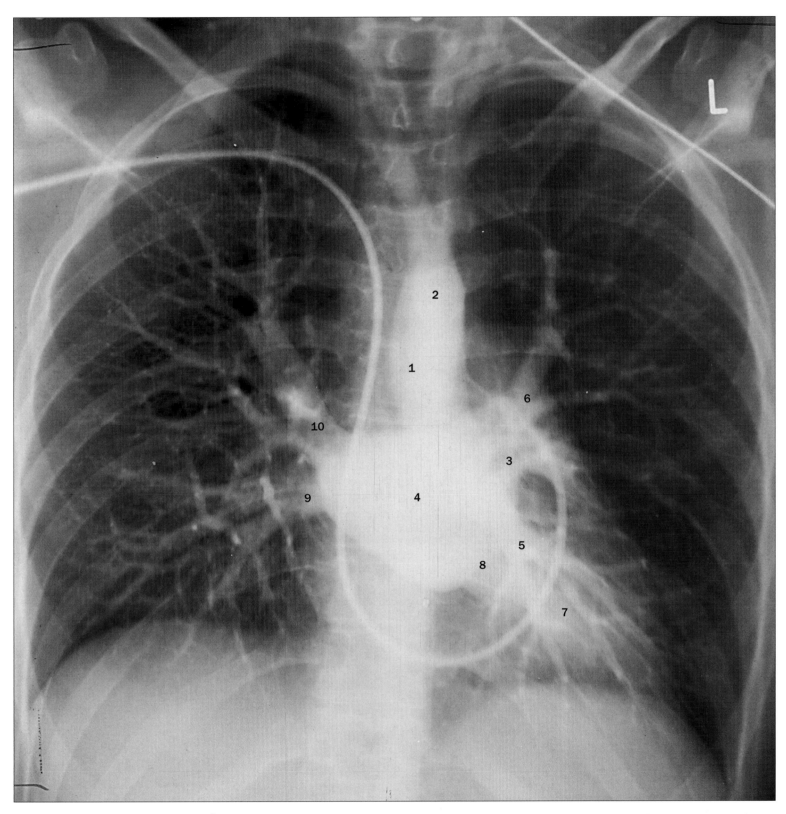

Pulmonary arteriogram – venous phase.

1 Aorta	**6** Left superior pulmonary vein
2 Aortic arch	**7** Left ventricle
3 Left atrial appendage (auricle)	**8** Mitral valve
4 Left atrium	**9** Right inferior pulmonary vein
5 Left inferior pulmonary vein	**10** Right superior pulmonary vein

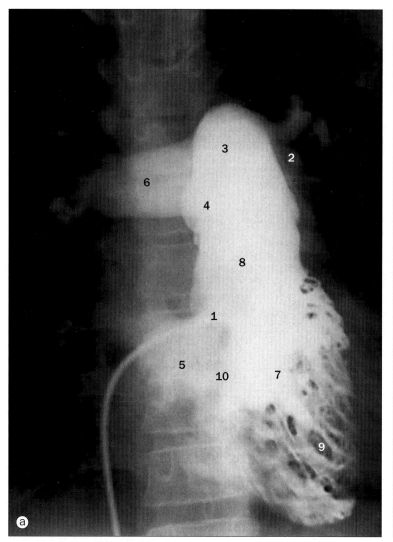
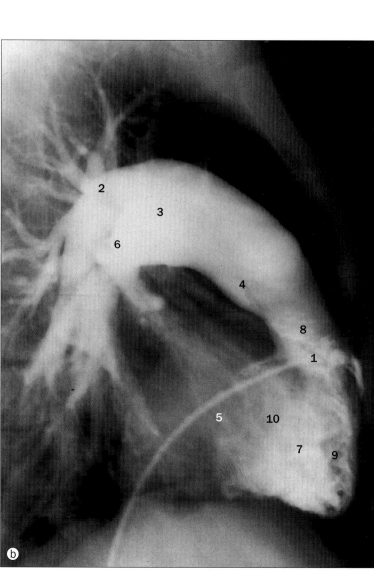

(a) and (b) Right ventricular angiograms.

 1 Catheter in right ventricle via inferior vena cava and right atrium
 2 Left main pulmonary artery
 3 Pulmonary artery
 4 Pulmonary valve
 5 Right atrium
 6 Right main pulmonary artery
 7 Right ventricle
 8 Right ventricular outflow tract
 9 Trabeculae of right ventricle
10 Tricuspid valve

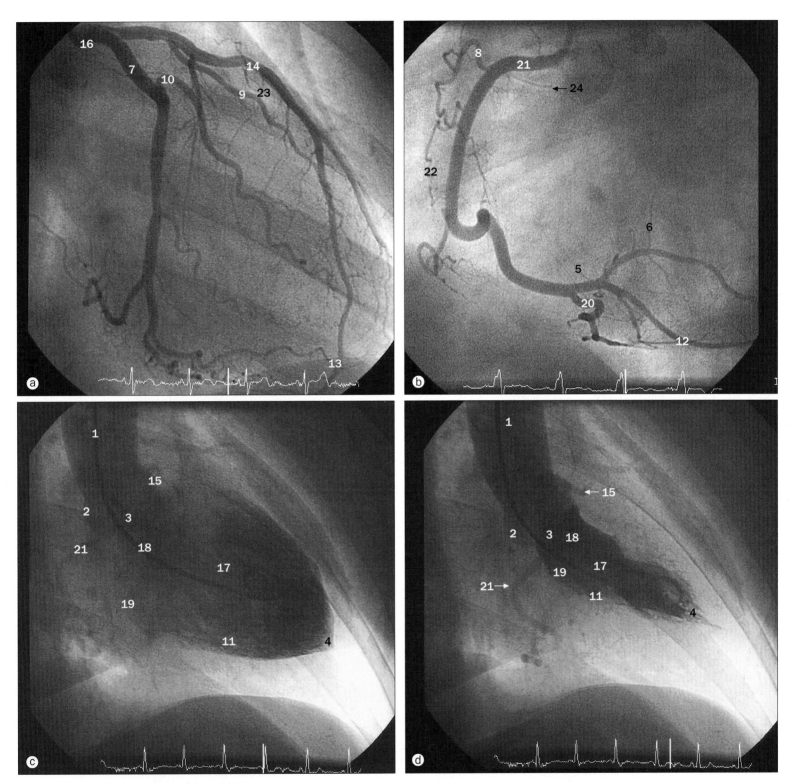

(a) Left coronary arteriogram, (b) right coronary arteriogram, (c) left ventricular angiogram, diastolic phase, (d) left ventricular angiogram, systolic phase.

1 Aorta	**10** First obtuse marginal branch of circumflex artery	**16** Left main stem coronary artery
2 Aortic sinus	**11** Inferior wall of left ventricle	**17** Left ventricular cavity
3 Aortic valve	**12** Lateral ventricular branch to left ventricle	**18** Left ventricular outflow tract
4 Apex of the left ventricle	**13** Left anterior interventricular artery curving round apex of heart	**19** Mitral valve
5 Atrioventricular nodal artery	**14** Left anterior interventricular branch (left anterior descending)	**20** Posterior interventricular septal artery (posterior descending artery)
6 Branch to left atrium	**15** Left coronary artery	**21** Right coronary artery
7 Circumflex artery		**22** Right marginal arteries
8 Conus artery		**23** Septal arteries
9 Diagonal arteries		**24** Sinuatrial nodal artery

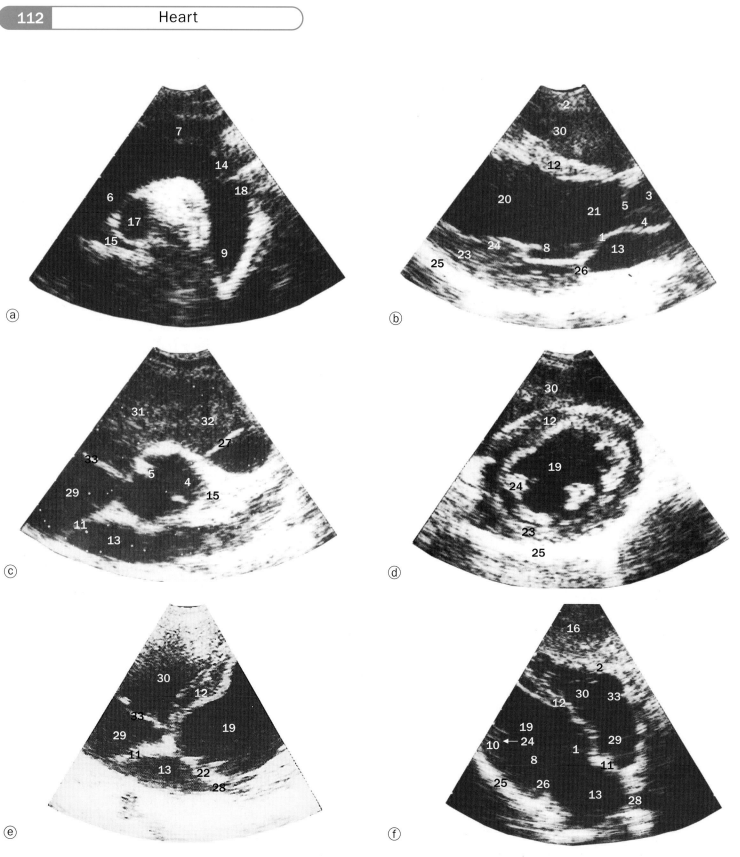

Heart, (a) suprasternal arch of aorta, (b) left parasternal long axis of left ventricle, (c) left parasternal short axis at aortic valve, (d) left parasternal short axis at papillary muscles, (e) apical four chamber, (f) subcostal four chamber. Ultrasound images.

1 Anterior leaflet of the mitral valve	**9** Descending aorta	**17** Left pulmonary artery	**26** Posterior leaflet of the mitral valve
2 Anterior wall of right ventricle	**10** Inferior wall of left ventricle	**18** Left subclavian artery	**27** Pulmonary valve
3 Aorta	**11** Interatrial septum	**19** Left ventricle	**28** Pulmonary vein
4 Aortic sinus	**12** Interventricular septum	**20** Left ventricular cavity	**29** Right atrium
5 Aortic valve	**13** Left atrium	**21** Left ventricular outflow tract	**30** Right ventricle
6 Ascending aorta	**14** Left common carotid artery	**22** Mitral valve	**31** Right ventricular cavity
7 Brachiocephalic trunk	**15** Left coronary artery	**23** Myocardium	**32** Right ventricular outflow tract
8 Chordae tendineae	**16** Left lobe of liver	**24** Papillary muscles	**33** Tricuspid valve
		25 Pericardium	

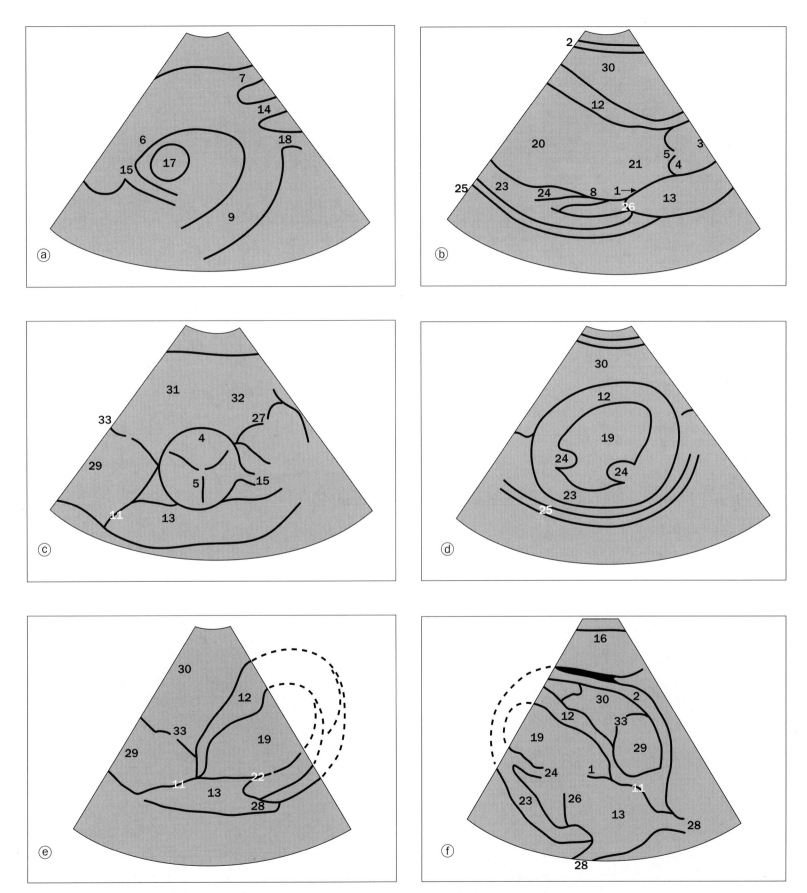

Line diagrams of the electrocardiographic images opposite. See page 112 for key.

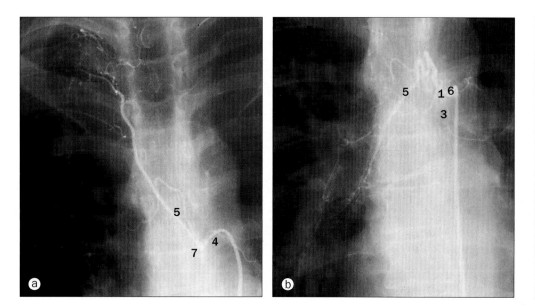

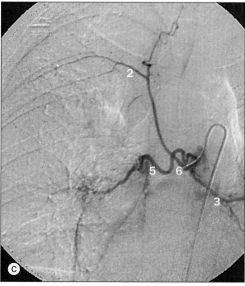

(a)–(c) Right bronchial arteriograms.

There is a great variability in the anatomy of the bronchial arteries, but the majority originate from the descending thoracic aorta, above the level of the left main stem bronchus between the upper border of the fifth thoracic vertebra and the lower border of the sixth thoracic vertebra. The number of bronchial arteries on each side may vary between one and four. Usually, there is one vessel to the right lung and two to the left. Accessory bronchial arteries may arise from the brachiocephalic artery and subclavian arteries, or from other branches such as the internal thoracic, pericardiophrenic and oesophageal arteries. In many cases the right bronchial artery arises from an intercostobronchial trunk, but in this example the trunk is very short and divides almost immediately into a right bronchial artery, which is directed towards the hilum, and the first right aortic intercostal artery. Reflux filling of the left bronchial artery is seen.
 A second larger bronchial artery which has been catheterised (b) has a common trunk arising from the front of the aorta, giving rise to a right and left bronchial artery.

1 Common bronchial trunk
2 Intercostal artery
3 Left bronchial branches
4 Reflux filling of left bronchial artery
5 Right bronchial artery
6 Tip of catheter in common bronchial arterial trunk
7 Tip of catheter in intercostobronchial trunk

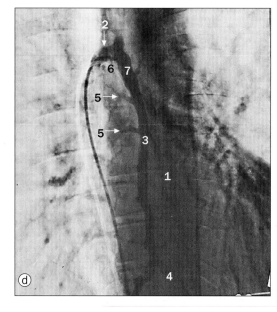

(d) Azygos venogram.

In the thorax the vertebral veins drain into intercostal veins, while in the lumbar region the lumbar veins drain into the ascending lumbar veins. The right ascending lumbar vein becomes the azygos vein on entering the thorax, and the left ascending lumbar vein becomes the hemi-azygos vein. At the level of the fourth thoracic vertebra, the azygos vein turns anteriorly (the arch of the azygos) to enter the superior vena cava. The hemi-azygos vein crosses to join the azygos vein at the level of the eighth or ninth thoracic vertebral body. The accessory hemi-azygos vein is continuous with the hemi-azygos vein inferiorly and the left superior intercostal vein superiorly.

1 Accessory hemi-azygos vein
2 Azygos arch
3 Azygos vein
4 Hemi-azygos vein
5 Intercostal veins
6 Subtraction artefact caused by cardiac and catheter movement
7 Tip of catheter introduced via femoral vein into superior vena cava and azygos vein

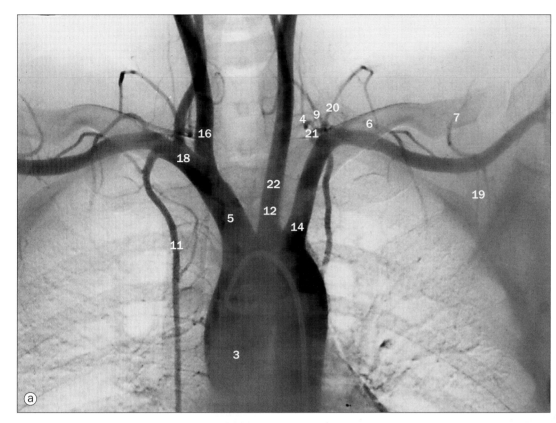

(a) Subtracted arch aortogram, anteroposterior image.
• The vertebral artery (22) has a separate origin off the arch, projected over the left common carotid artery in this view. This is a normal variant.

(b) Subtracted arch aortogram, left anterior oblique image. The origins of the supra-aortic branches are best shown by left anterior oblique projection, so that the origins of the vessels are not superimposed. There are many congenital variations in the way in which the major vessels arise from the aortic arch, but the most common is shown in (b).

(c) Left ventricular angiogram.

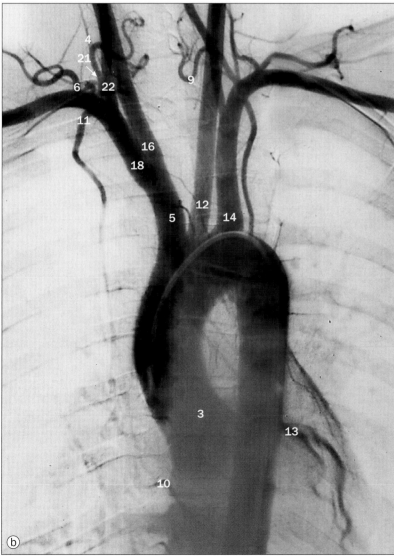

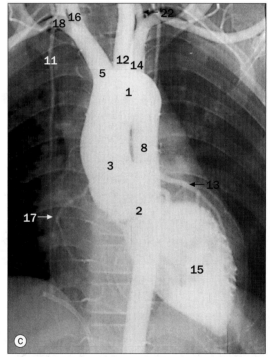

1 Aortic arch	**12** Left common carotid artery
2 Aortic valve	**13** Left coronary artery
3 Ascending aorta	**14** Left subclavian artery
4 Ascending cervical artery	**15** Left ventricle
5 Brachiocephalic trunk	**16** Right common carotid artery
6 Costocervical trunk	
7 Deltoid branch of thoraco-acromial artery	**17** Right coronary artery
	18 Right subclavian artery
8 Descending aorta	**19** Superior thoracic artery
9 Inferior thyroid artery	**20** Suprascapular artery
10 Intercostal artery	**21** Thyrocervical trunk
11 Internal thoracic artery	**22** Vertebral artery

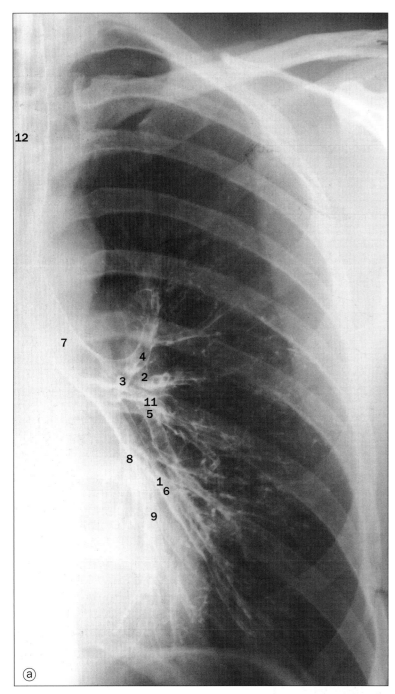

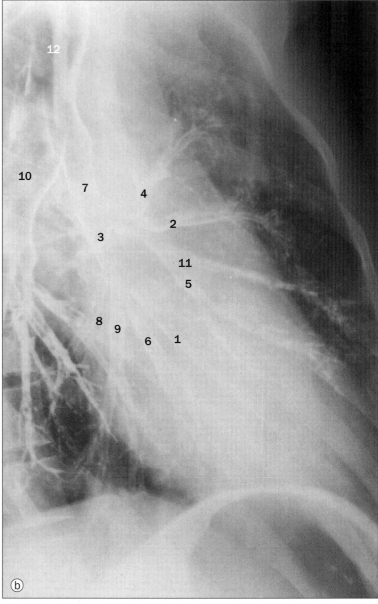

Left lung bronchogram, (**a**) postero-anterior image, (**b**) oblique projection.

1 Anterior basal segmental bronchus
2 Anterior segmental bronchus
3 Apical (superior) segmental bronchus
4 Apicoposterior segmental bronchus
5 Inferior lingular segmental bronchus
6 Lateral basal segmental bronchus
7 Left main bronchus
8 Medial basal segmental bronchus
9 Posterior basal segmental bronchus
10 Right main bronchus
11 Superior lingular segmental bronchus
12 Trachea

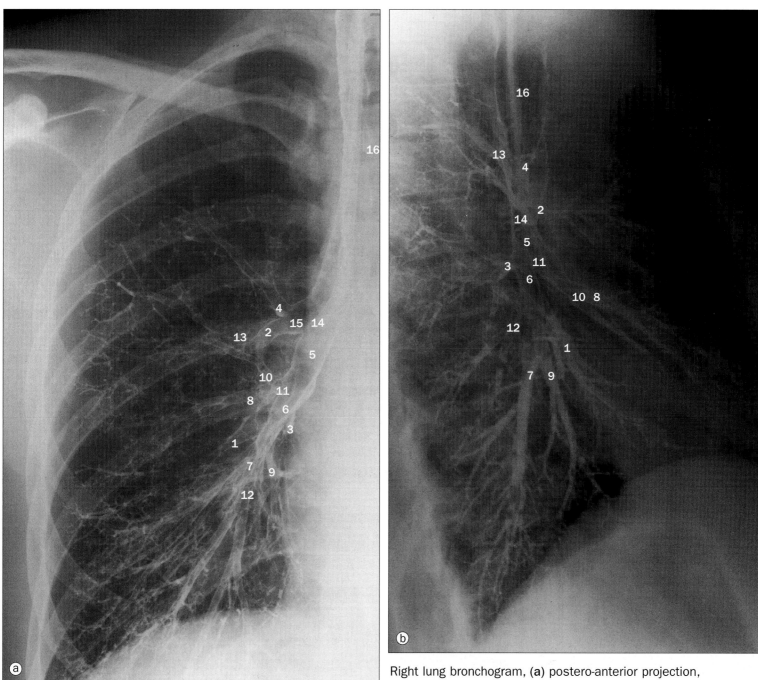

Right lung bronchogram, (a) postero-anterior projection, (b) lateral projection.

1 Anterior basal segmental bronchus
2 Anterior segmental bronchus
3 Apical (superior) segmental bronchus
4 Apical segmental bronchus
5 Bronchus intermedius
6 Inferior lobe bronchus
7 Lateral basal segmental bronchus
8 Lateral segmental bronchus of middle lobe
9 Medial basal segmental bronchus
10 Medial segmental bronchus of middle lobe
11 Middle lobe bronchus
12 Posterior basal segmental bronchus
13 Posterior segmental bronchus
14 Right main bronchus
15 Right superior lobe bronchus
16 Trachea

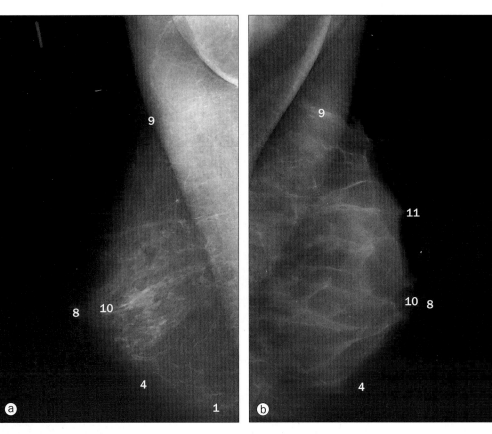

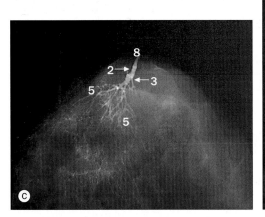

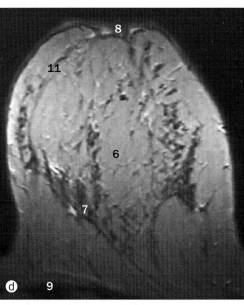

1	Inframammary fold
2	Lactiferous duct
3	Lactiferous sinus
4	Line of skin
5	Lobar duct pattern (comprising (intra) lobar ducts and terminal ductal lobular units)
6	Mammary fat
7	Mammary fibroglandular tissue
8	Nipple
9	Pectoral muscle
10	Subareolar area
11	Suspensory ligament (Cooper's)

(a) Postmenopausal right breast, mediolateral oblique mammogram.

(b) Premenopausal left breast, lateral oblique mammogram.

(c) Premenopausal right breast, craniocaudal image from a ductogram.

(d) Mammogram, MR image.

5 | Abdomen

Abdomen, supine projection.

1 Gas in caecum and
  ascending colon
2 Gas in descending colon
3 Gas in stomach
4 Left kidney
5 Left psoas muscle
6 Right kidney
7 Right psoas muscle
8 Twelfth rib

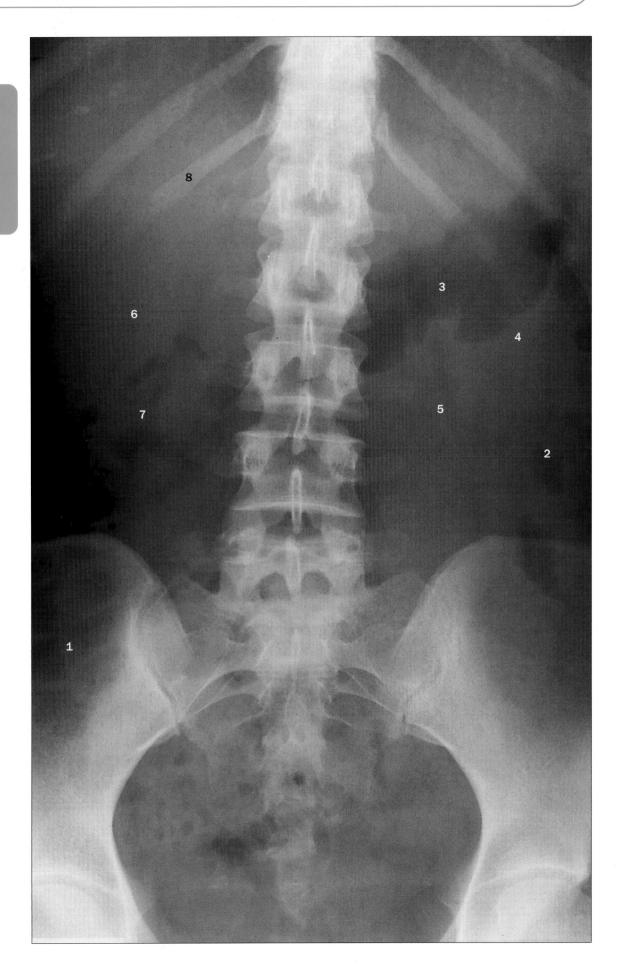

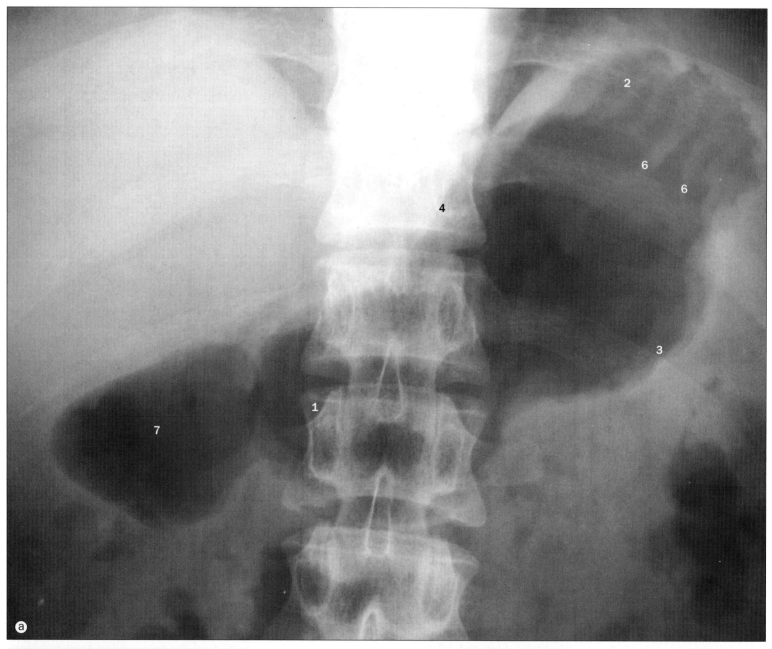

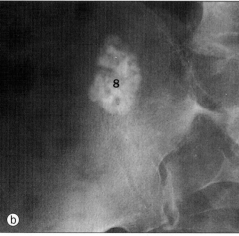

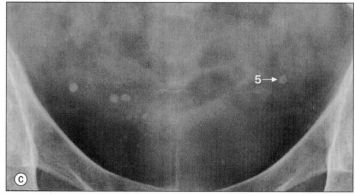

Abdomen, **(a)** demonstrating gas in stomach and first part of duodenum, **(b)** demonstrating a calcified lymph node, **(c)** demonstrating calcified pelvic veins (phleboliths), supine projections.

1 Antrum of stomach
2 Fundus
3 Greater curvature of stomach
4 Lesser curvature of stomach
5 Phlebolith
6 Rugae of stomach
7 Superior (first) part of duodenum (duodenal cap)
8 Calcified lymph mode

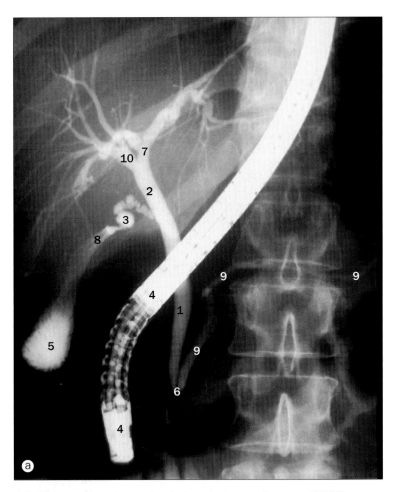

(a) Endoscopic retrograde cholangiopancreatogram (ERCP).

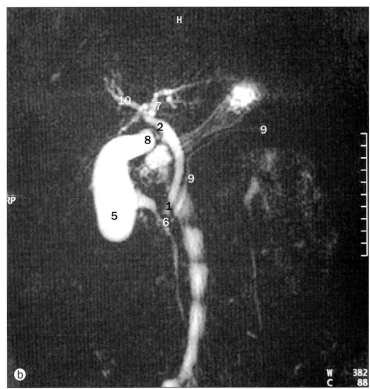

(b) Magnetic cholangiopancreatogram (MRCP).

1	Common bile duct	**5**	Gall bladder	**8**	Neck of gall bladder
2	Common hepatic duct	**6**	Hepatopancreatic (Vater's) ampulla	**9**	Pancreatic duct
3	Cystic duct	**7**	Left hepatic duct	**10**	Right hepatic duct
4	Endoscope in duodenum				

1 Accessory pancreatic duct (Santorini's)
2 Ampullary part of pancreatic duct
3 Common bile duct
4 Contrast and gas in descending (second) part of duodenum
5 Intralobular ducts
6 Main pancreatic duct

(c) ERCP

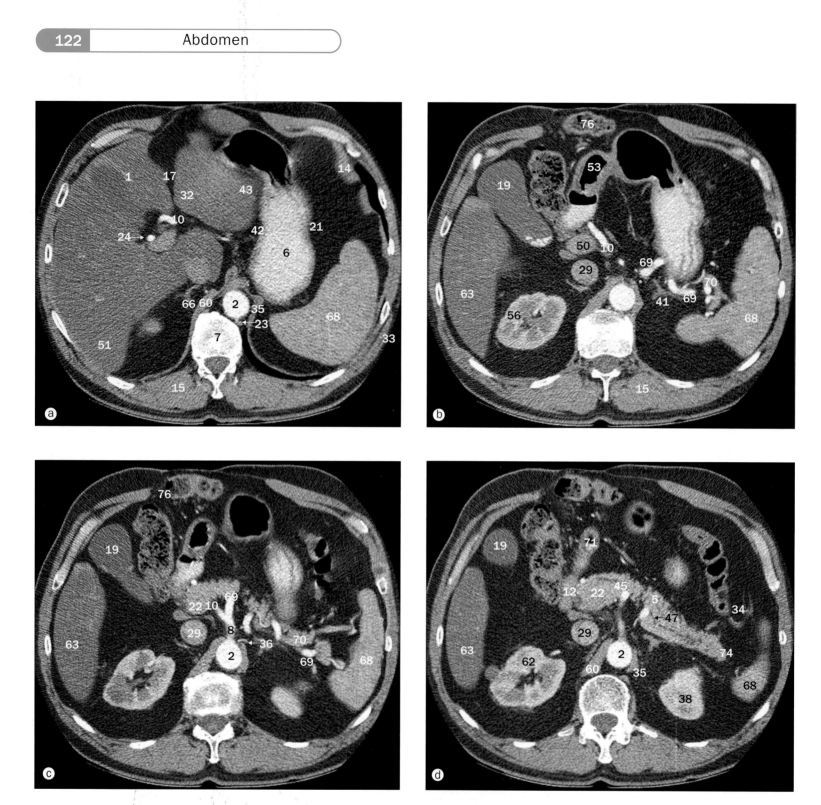

The following eight axial CT images (a–h) of the upper abdomen are taken during the arterial phase of a contrast injection to demonstrate the arterial system. The same patient's venous anatomy is demonstrated immediately following these images (i–t).

1 Anterior segment of right lobe of liver	**14** Diaphragm	**27** Ilium
2 Aorta	**15** Erector spinae muscle	**28** Inferior mesenteric artery
3 Ascending colon	**16** External oblique muscle	**29** Inferior vena cava
4 Azygos vein	**17** Fissure for ligamentum venosum	**30** Internal oblique muscle
5 Body of pancreas	**18** Fundus of stomach	**31** Jejunum
6 Body of stomach	**19** Gall bladder	**32** Lateral segment of left lobe of liver
7 Body of vertebra	**20** Gluteus medius muscle	**33** Latissimus dorsi muscle
8 Coeliac trunk	**21** Greater curvature of stomach	**34** Left colic (splenic) flexure
9 Common bile duct	**22** Head of pancreas	**35** Left crus of diaphragm
10 Common hepatic artery	**23** Hemi-azygos vein	**36** Left gastric artery
11 Common iliac artery	**24** Hepatic artery	**37** Left hepatic vein
12 Descending (second) part of duodenum	**25** Horizontal (third) part of duodenum	**38** Left kidney
13 Descending colon	**26** Ileum	**39** Left renal artery

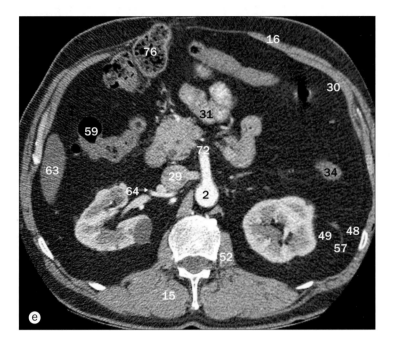

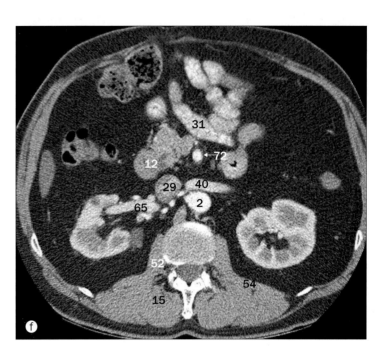

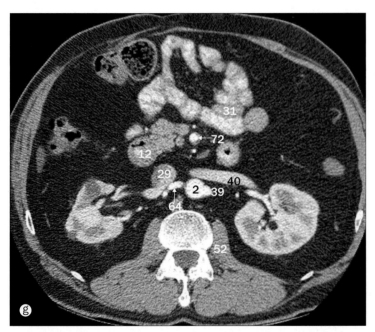

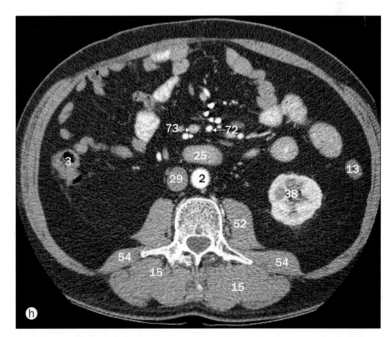

40 Left renal vein	53 Pyloric part of stomach	66 Right suprarenal gland
41 Left suprarenal gland	54 Quadratus lumborum muscle	67 Serratus anterior muscle
42 Lesser curvature of stomach	55 Rectus abdominis muscle	68 Spleen
43 Medial segment of left lobe of liver	56 Renal cortex	69 Splenic artery
44 Middle hepatic vein	57 Renal fascia	70 Splenic vein
45 Neck of pancreas	58 Renal pelvis	71 Superior (first) part of duodenum
46 Oesophagus	59 Right colic (hepatic) flexure	72 Superior mesenteric artery
47 Pancreatic duct	60 Right crus of diaphragm	73 Superior mesenteric vein
48 Pararenal fat	61 Right hepatic vein	74 Tail of pancreas
49 Perirenal fat	62 Right kidney	75 Thecal sac
50 Portal vein	63 Right lobe of liver	76 Transverse colon
51 Posterior segment of right lobe of liver	64 Right renal artery	
52 Psoas major muscle	65 Right renal vein	

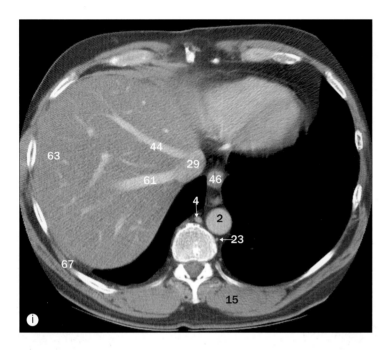

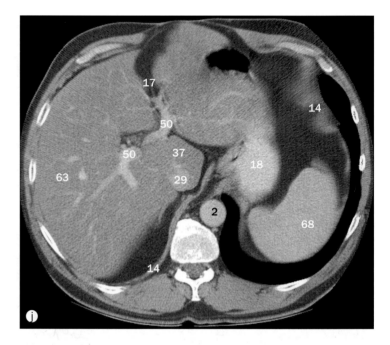

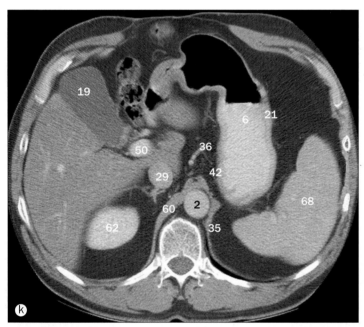

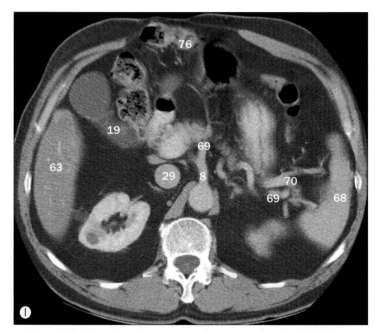

(i)–(l) Axial CT scans through the abdomen taken during the venous phase of a contrast injection. The patient's arterial phase examinations are in the immediately preceding section.

1 Anterior segment of right lobe of liver	**15** Erector spinae muscle	**29** Inferior vena cava
2 Aorta	**16** External oblique muscle	**30** Internal oblique muscle
3 Ascending colon	**17** Fissure for ligamentum venosum	**31** Jejunum
4 Azygos vein	**18** Fundus of stomach	**32** Lateral segment of left lobe of liver
5 Body of pancreas	**19** Gall bladder	**33** Latissimus dorsi muscle
6 Body of stomach	**20** Gluteus medius muscle	**34** Left colic (splenic) flexure
7 Body of vertebra	**21** Greater curvature of stomach	**35** Left crus of diaphragm
8 Coeliac trunk	**22** Head of pancreas	**36** Left gastric artery
9 Common bile duct	**23** Hemi-azygos vein	**37** Left hepatic vein
10 Common hepatic artery	**24** Hepatic artery	**38** Left kidney
11 Common iliac artery	**25** Horizontal (third) part of duodenum	**39** Left renal artery
12 Descending (second) part of duodenum	**26** Ileum	**40** Left renal vein
13 Descending colon	**27** Ilium	**41** Left suprarenal gland
14 Diaphragm	**28** Inferior mesenteric artery	**42** Lesser curvature of stomach

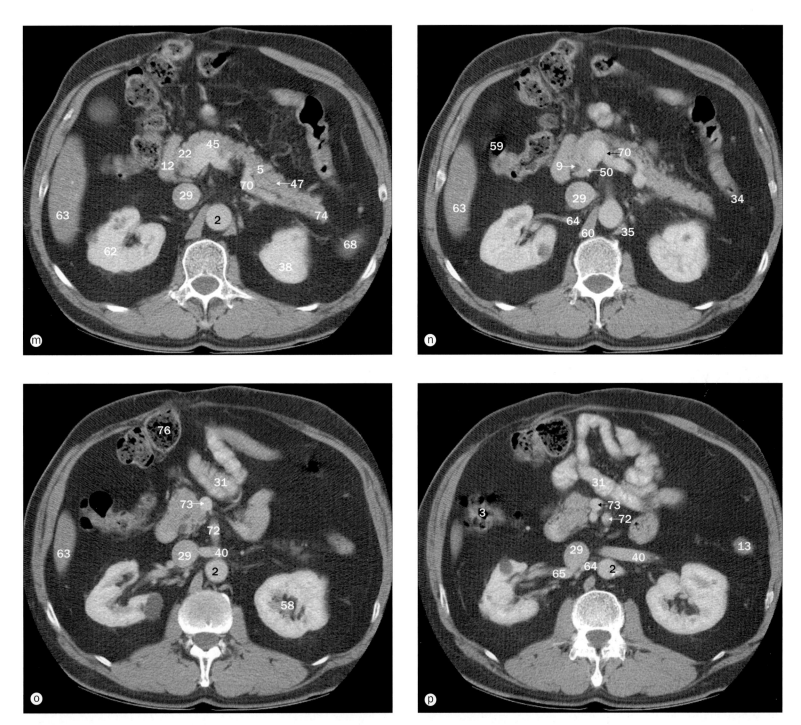

(m)–(p) Axial CT scans through the abdomen taken during the venous phase of a contrast injection.

43 Medial segment of left lobe of liver	**55** Rectus abdominis muscle	**67** Serratus anterior muscle
44 Middle hepatic vein	**56** Renal cortex	**68** Spleen
45 Neck of pancreas	**57** Renal fascia	**69** Splenic artery
46 Oesophagus	**58** Renal pelvis	**70** Splenic vein
47 Pancreatic duct	**59** Right colic (hepatic) flexure	**71** Superior (first) part of duodenum
48 Pararenal fat	**60** Right crus of diaphragm	**72** Superior mesenteric artery
49 Perirenal fat	**61** Right hepatic vein	**73** Superior mesenteric vein
50 Portal vein	**62** Right kidney	**74** Tail of pancreas
51 Posterior segment of right lobe of liver	**63** Right lobe of liver	**75** Thecal sac
52 Psoas major muscle	**64** Right renal artery	**76** Transverse colon
53 Pyloric part of stomach	**65** Right renal vein	
54 Quadratus lumborum muscle	**66** Right suprarenal gland	

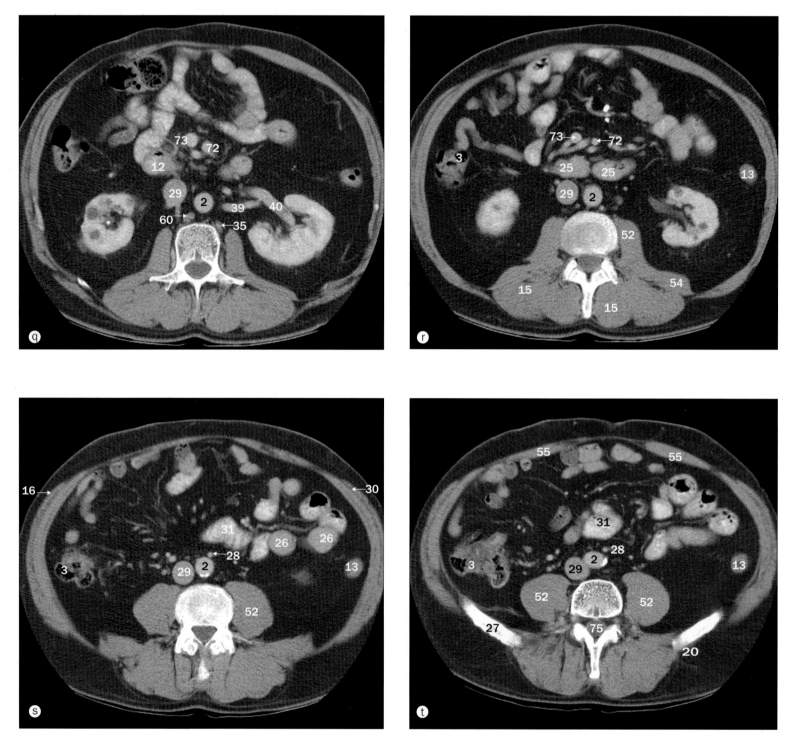

(q)–(t) Axial CT scans through the abdomen taken during the venous phase of a contrast injection.

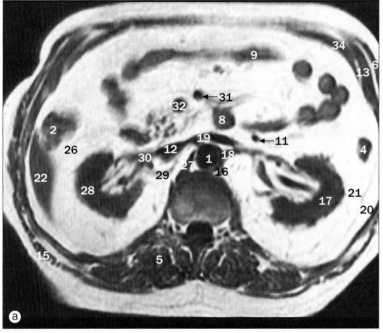

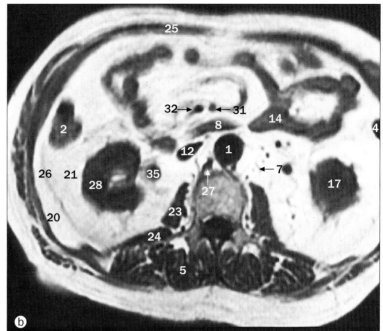

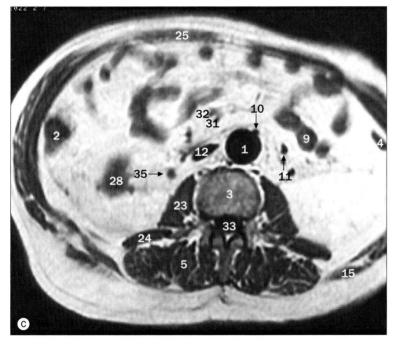

(a)–(f) Abdomen, axial MR images.

1	Aorta	19	Left renal vein
2	Ascending colon	20	Pararenal fat
3	Body of vertebra	21	Perirenal fat
4	Descending colon	22	Posterior segment of right
5	Erector spinae muscle		lobe of liver
6	External oblique muscle	23	Psoas major muscle
7	Gonadal artery and vein	24	Quadratus lumborum muscle
8	Horizontal (third) part of	25	Rectus abdominis muscle
	duodenum	26	Renal fascia
9	Ileum	27	Right crus of diaphragm
10	Inferior mesenteric artery	28	Right kidney
11	Inferior mesenteric vein	29	Right renal artery
12	Inferior vena cava	30	Right renal vein
13	Internal oblique muscle	31	Superior mesenteric artery
14	Jejunum	32	Superior mesenteric vein
15	Latissimus dorsi muscle	33	Thecal sac
16	Left crus of diaphragm	34	Transversus abdominis
17	Left kidney		muscle
18	Left renal artery	35	Ureter

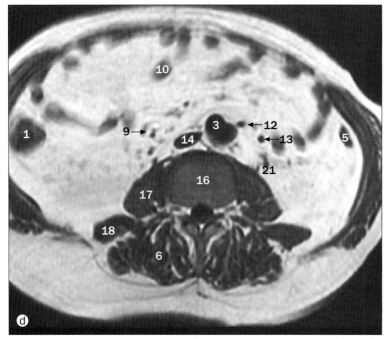

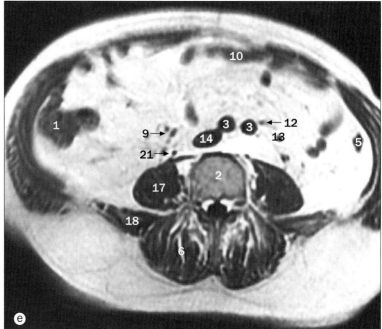

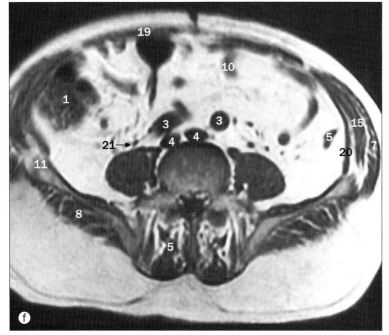

(d)–(f) Abdomen, axial MR images.

1	Ascending colon	**12**	Inferior mesenteric artery
2	Body of vertebra	**13**	Inferior mesenteric vein
3	Common iliac artery	**14**	Inferior vena cava
4	Common iliac vein	**15**	Internal oblique muscle
5	Descending colon	**16**	Intervertebral disc
6	Erector spinae muscle	**17**	Psoas major muscle
7	External oblique muscle	**18**	Quadratus lumborum muscle
8	Gluteus medius muscle	**19**	Rectus abdominis muscle
9	Gonadal artery and vein	**20**	Transversus abdominis
10	Ileum		muscle
11	Ilium	**21**	Ureter

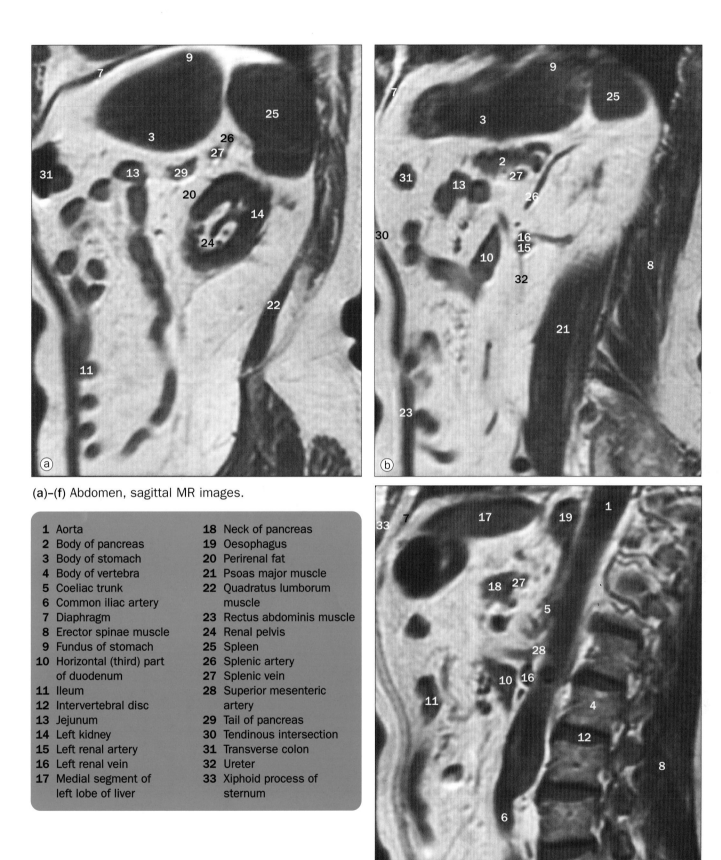

(a)–(f) Abdomen, sagittal MR images.

1 Aorta	**18** Neck of pancreas
2 Body of pancreas	**19** Oesophagus
3 Body of stomach	**20** Perirenal fat
4 Body of vertebra	**21** Psoas major muscle
5 Coeliac trunk	**22** Quadratus lumborum
6 Common iliac artery	muscle
7 Diaphragm	**23** Rectus abdominis muscle
8 Erector spinae muscle	**24** Renal pelvis
9 Fundus of stomach	**25** Spleen
10 Horizontal (third) part	**26** Splenic artery
of duodenum	**27** Splenic vein
11 Ileum	**28** Superior mesenteric
12 Intervertebral disc	artery
13 Jejunum	**29** Tail of pancreas
14 Left kidney	**30** Tendinous intersection
15 Left renal artery	**31** Transverse colon
16 Left renal vein	**32** Ureter
17 Medial segment of	**33** Xiphoid process of
left lobe of liver	sternum

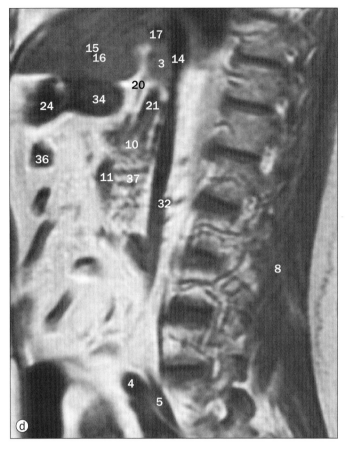

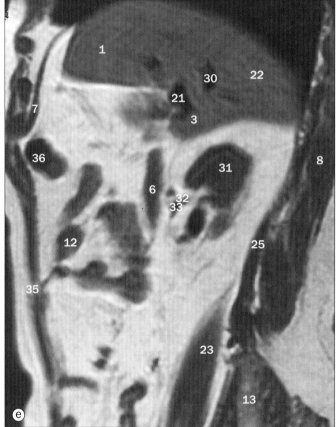

(d)–(f) Abdomen, sagittal MR images.

1 Anterior segment of right lobe of liver	**20** Porta hepatis
2 Ascending colon	**21** Portal vein
3 Caudate lobe of liver	**22** Posterior segment of right lobe of liver
4 Common iliac artery	**23** Psoas major muscle
5 Common iliac vein	**24** Pyloric part of stomach
6 Descending (second) part of duodenum	**25** Quadratus lumborum muscle
7 Diaphragm	**26** Rectus abdominis muscle
8 Erector spinae muscle	**27** Renal fascia
9 Gall bladder	**28** Renal pelvis
10 Head of pancreas	**29** Right colic (hepatic) flexure
11 Horizontal (third) part of duodenum	**30** Right hepatic vein
12 Ileum	**31** Right kidney
13 Ilium	**32** Right renal artery
14 Inferior vena cava	**33** Right renal vein
15 Lateral segment of left lobe of liver	**34** Superior (first) part of duodenum
16 Left hepatic vein	**35** Tendinous intersection
17 Middle hepatic vein	**36** Transverse colon
18 Pararenal fat	**37** Uncinate process of head of pancreas
19 Perirenal fat	

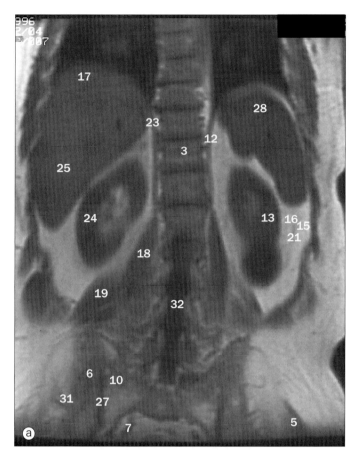

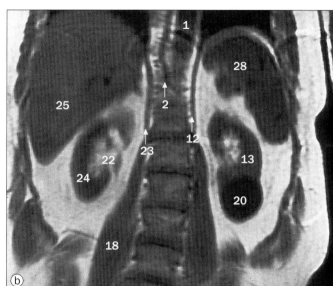

(a)–(f) Abdomen, coronal MR images.
• Note the small left renal cyst.

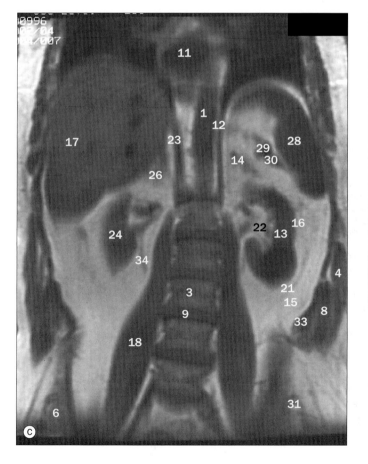

1 Aorta	**18** Psoas major muscle
2 Azygos vein	**19** Quadratus lumborum
3 Body of vertebra	muscle
4 External oblique muscle	**20** Renal cyst
5 Gluteus maximus muscle	**21** Renal fascia
6 Ilium	**22** Renal pelvis
7 Internal iliac artery	**23** Right crus of diaphragm
8 Internal oblique muscle	**24** Right kidney
9 Intervertebral disc	**25** Right lobe of liver
10 Lateral part (ala) of	**26** Right suprarenal gland
sacrum	**27** Sacro-iliac joint
11 Left atrium	**28** Spleen
12 Left crus of diaphragm	**29** Splenic artery
13 Left kidney	**30** Splenic vein
14 Left suprarenal gland	**31** Superior gluteal artery
15 Pararenal fat	**32** Thecal sac
16 Perirenal fat	**33** Transversus abdominis
17 Posterior segment of	muscle
right lobe of liver	**34** Ureter

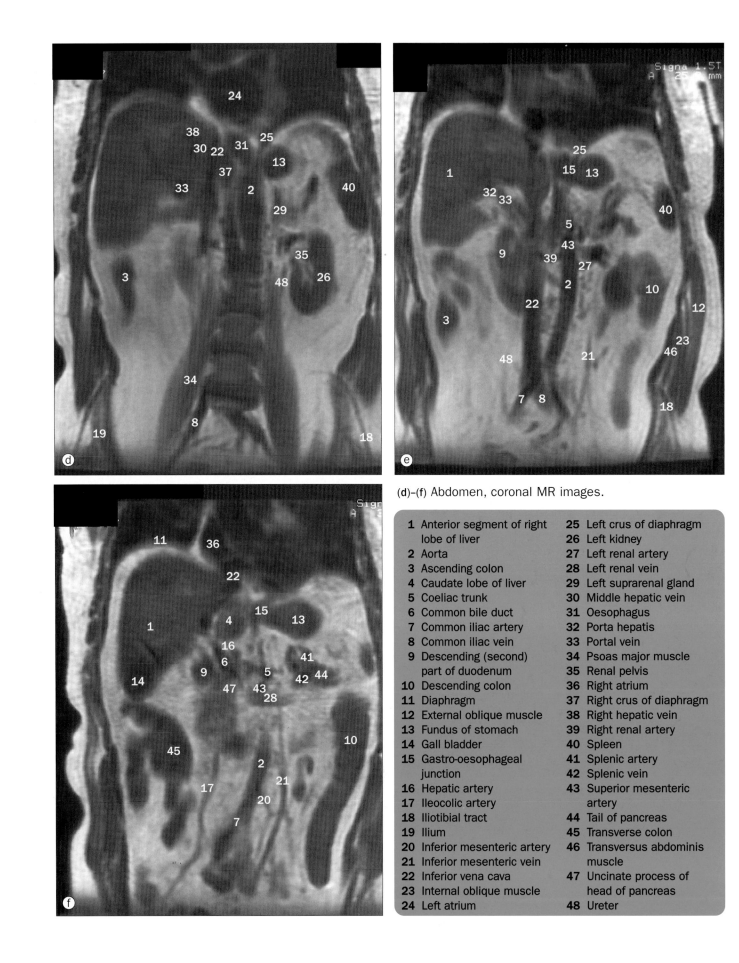

(d)–(f) Abdomen, coronal MR images.

1	Anterior segment of right lobe of liver	25	Left crus of diaphragm
		26	Left kidney
2	Aorta	27	Left renal artery
3	Ascending colon	28	Left renal vein
4	Caudate lobe of liver	29	Left suprarenal gland
5	Coeliac trunk	30	Middle hepatic vein
6	Common bile duct	31	Oesophagus
7	Common iliac artery	32	Porta hepatis
8	Common iliac vein	33	Portal vein
9	Descending (second) part of duodenum	34	Psoas major muscle
		35	Renal pelvis
10	Descending colon	36	Right atrium
11	Diaphragm	37	Right crus of diaphragm
12	External oblique muscle	38	Right hepatic vein
13	Fundus of stomach	39	Right renal artery
14	Gall bladder	40	Spleen
15	Gastro-oesophageal junction	41	Splenic artery
		42	Splenic vein
16	Hepatic artery	43	Superior mesenteric artery
17	Ileocolic artery		
18	Iliotibial tract	44	Tail of pancreas
19	Ilium	45	Transverse colon
20	Inferior mesenteric artery	46	Transversus abdominis muscle
21	Inferior mesenteric vein		
22	Inferior vena cava	47	Uncinate process of head of pancreas
23	Internal oblique muscle		
24	Left atrium	48	Ureter

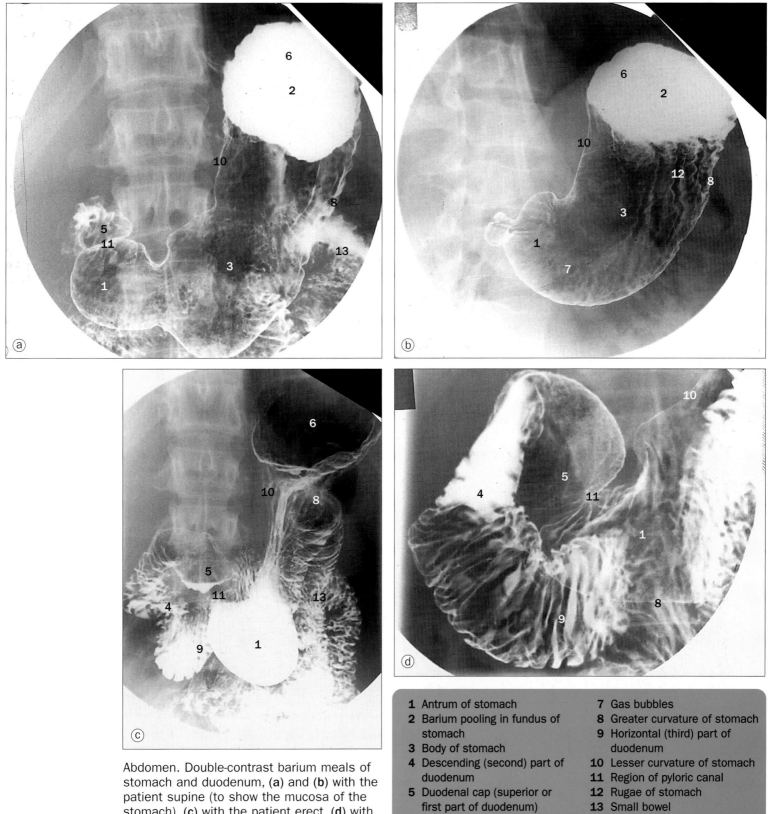

Abdomen. Double-contrast barium meals of stomach and duodenum, **(a)** and **(b)** with the patient supine (to show the mucosa of the stomach), **(c)** with the patient erect, **(d)** with the patient in a supine oblique position (to show the duodenum).

1 Antrum of stomach
2 Barium pooling in fundus of stomach
3 Body of stomach
4 Descending (second) part of duodenum
5 Duodenal cap (superior or first part of duodenum)
6 Fundus of stomach
7 Gas bubbles
8 Greater curvature of stomach
9 Horizontal (third) part of duodenum
10 Lesser curvature of stomach
11 Region of pyloric canal
12 Rugae of stomach
13 Small bowel

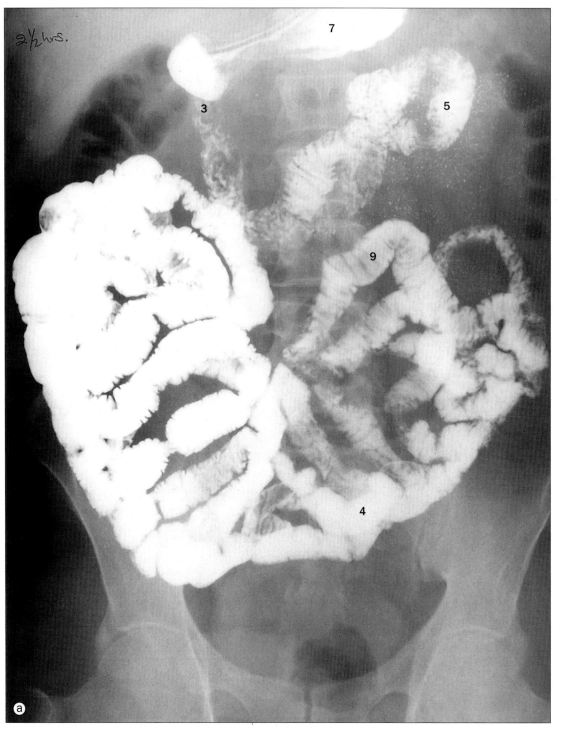

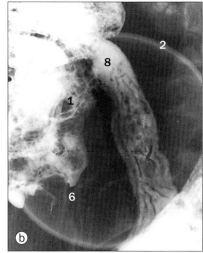

Abdomen, barium follow-throughs, (a) with the patient supine, (b) showing a localised view of the terminal ileum, anteroposterior radiographs.

1 Caecum	**6** Right sacro-iliac joint
2 Compression device	**7** Stomach
3 Descending (second) part of duodenum	**8** Terminal ileum
4 Proximal ileum	**9** Valvulae conniventes (plicae circulares)
5 Proximal jejunum	of jejunum

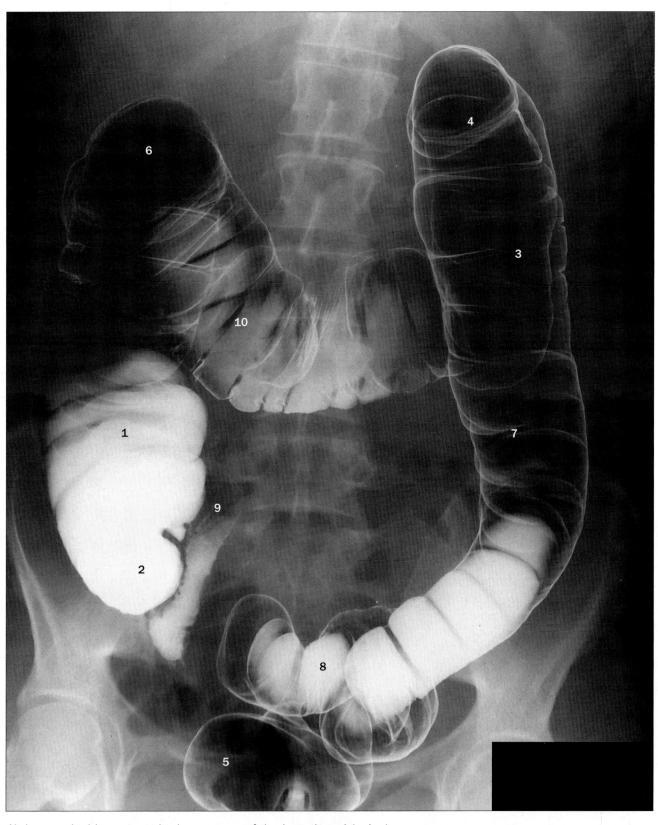

Abdomen, double-contrast barium enema of the large bowel (colon).

1	Ascending portion of colon	**6**	Right colic (hepatic) flexure of colon
2	Caecum	**7**	Sacculations (haustrations) of colon
3	Descending portion of colon	**8**	Sigmoid colon
4	Left colic (splenic) flexure of colon	**9**	Terminal ileum
5	Rectum	**10**	Transverse portion of colon

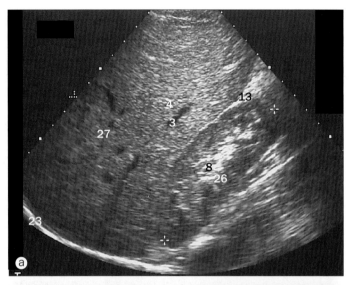
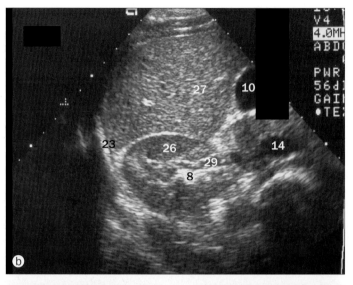
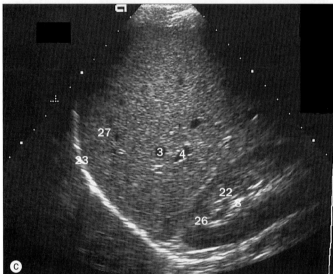
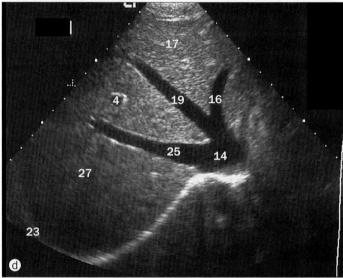
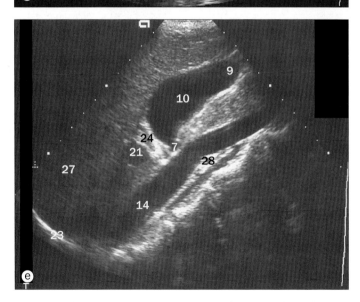
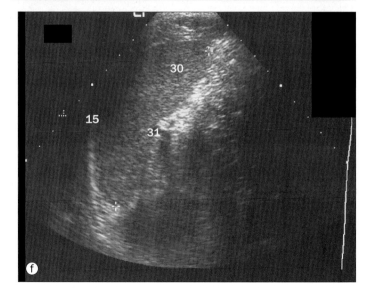

Abdominal ultrasound, (a)–(f) sagittal and parasagittal views.

1 Abdominal aorta	**6** Common bile duct	**11** Head of pancreas
2 Body of pancreas	**7** Cystic duct	**12** Hepatic artery
3 Branch of hepatic vein	**8** Fat in renal sinus	**13** Hepatorenal recess
4 Branch of portal vein	**9** Fundus of gall bladder	**14** Inferior vena cava
5 Coeliac trunk	**10** Gall bladder	**15** Left dome of diaphragm

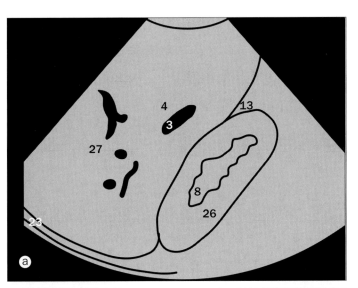

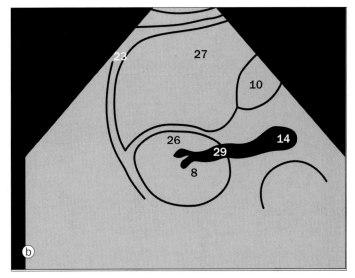

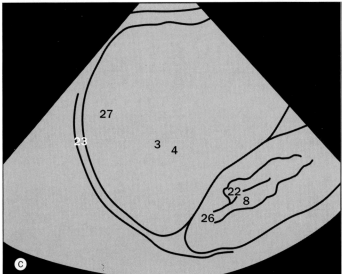

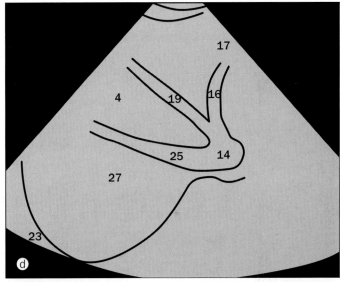

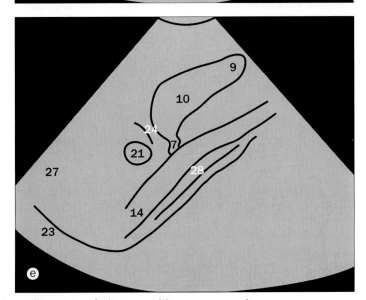

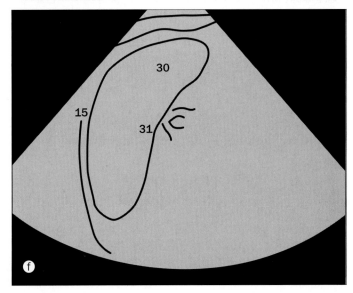

Line diagrams of ultrasound images opposite.

16	Left hepatic vein	**23**	Right dome of diaphragm	**30**	Spleen
17	Left lobe of liver	**24**	Right hepatic artery	**31**	Splenic vein
18	Left renal vein	**25**	Right hepatic vein	**32**	Superior mesenteric artery
19	Middle hepatic vein	**26**	Right kidney	**33**	Superior mesenteric vein
20	Neck of pancreas	**27**	Right lobe of liver	**34**	Tail of pancreas
21	Portal vein	**28**	Right renal artery	**35**	Vertebral body
22	Renal papilla	**29**	Right renal vein		

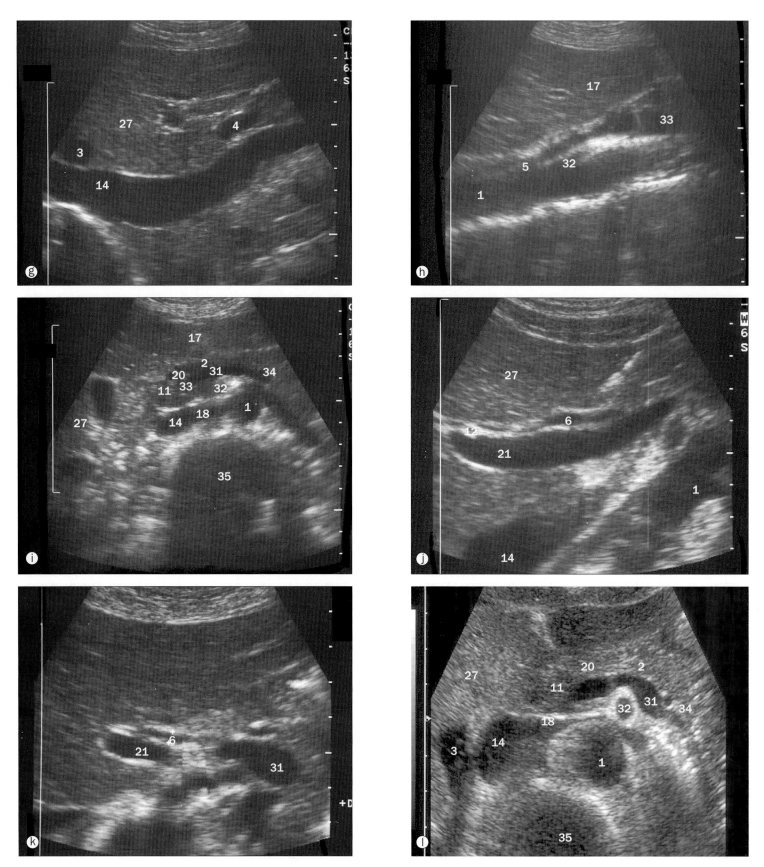

Abdominal ultrasound, (g)–(h) sagittal, (i)–(l) transverse and transverse oblique views.

1 Abdominal aorta	6 Common bile duct	11 Head of pancreas
2 Body of pancreas	7 Cystic duct	12 Hepatic artery
3 Branch of hepatic vein	8 Fat in renal sinus	13 Hepatorenal recess
4 Branch of portal vein	9 Fundus of gall bladder	14 Inferior vena cava
5 Coeliac trunk	10 Gall bladder	15 Left dome of diaphragm

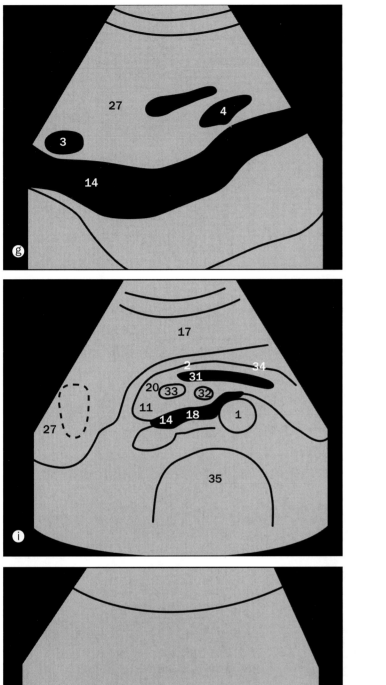

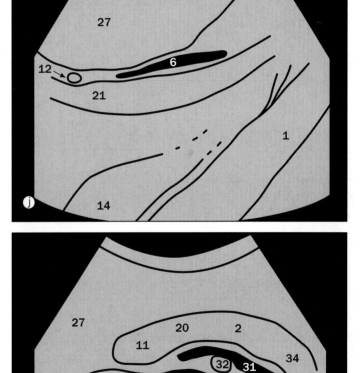

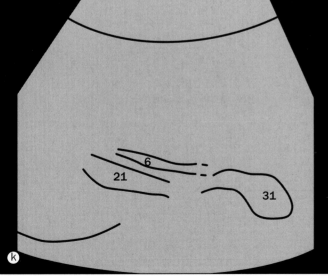

Line diagrams of ultrasound images opposite.

16 Left hepatic vein	**23** Right dome of diaphragm	**30** Spleen
17 Left lobe of liver	**24** Right hepatic artery	**31** Splenic vein
18 Left renal vein	**25** Right hepatic vein	**32** Superior mesenteric artery
19 Middle hepatic vein	**26** Right kidney	**33** Superior mesenteric vein
20 Neck of pancreas	**27** Right lobe of liver	**34** Tail of pancreas
21 Portal vein	**28** Right renal artery	**35** Vertebral body
22 Renal papilla	**29** Right renal vein	

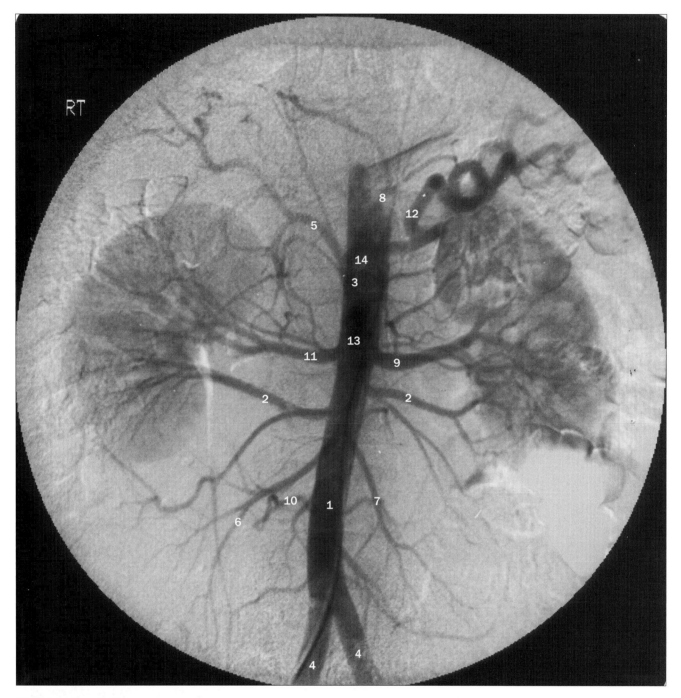

Abdominal aortogram.

1 Abdominal aorta
2 Accessory renal arteries
3 Coeliac trunk
4 Common iliac arteries
5 Hepatic artery
6 Ileocolic artery
7 Jejunal branches of superior mesenteric artery
8 Left gastric artery
9 Left renal artery
10 Lumbar arteries
11 Right renal artery
12 Splenic artery
13 Superior mesenteric artery
14 Tip of pigtail catheter in abdominal aorta

(a) and (b) Subtracted coeliac trunk arteriograms.

1 Dorsal pancreatic artery
2 Gastroduodenal artery
3 Hepatic artery
4 Left gastric artery
5 Left gastro-epiploic artery
6 Left hepatic artery
7 Pancreatica magna artery
8 Phrenic artery
9 Right gastro-epiploic artery
10 Right hepatic artery
11 Splenic artery
12 Superior pancreatico-duodenal artery
13 Tip of catheter in coeliac trunk
14 Transverse pancreatic artery

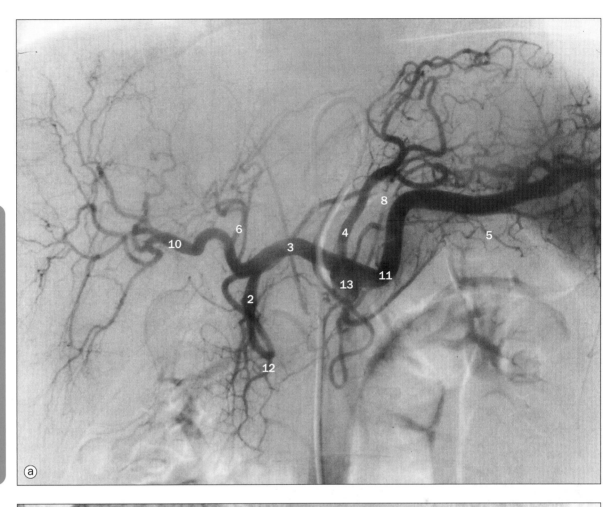

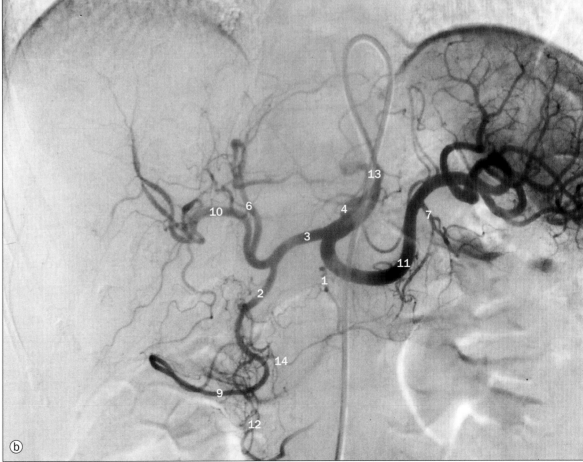

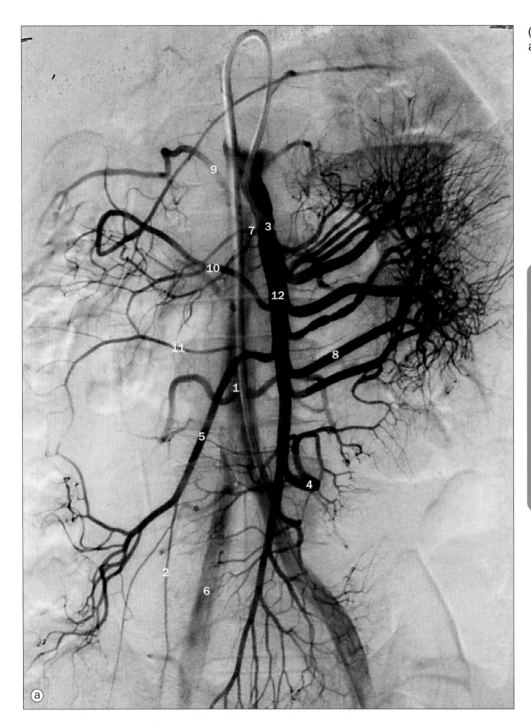

(a) Subtracted superior mesenteric arteriogram.

1 Aorta
2 Appendicular artery
3 Catheter with tip selectively in superior mesenteric artery
4 Ileal branches of superior mesenteric artery
5 Ileocolic artery
6 Iliac artery
7 Inferior pancreaticoduodenal artery
8 Jejunal branches of superior mesenteric artery
9 Lumbar arteries arising from abdominal aorta
10 Middle colic artery
11 Right colic artery
12 Superior mesenteric artery

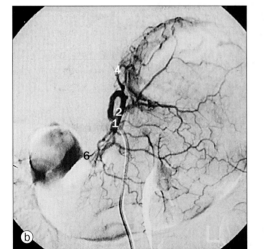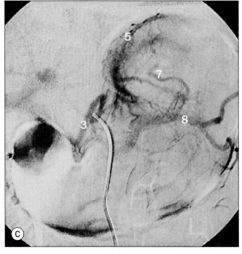

(b) Gastric arteries, (c) gastric veins.

1 Catheter in origin of left gastric artery
2 Left gastric artery
3 Left gastric vein
4 Oesophageal branch of left gastric artery
5 Oesophageal branches of left gastric vein
6 Right gastric artery
7 Short gastric veins
8 Splenic vein

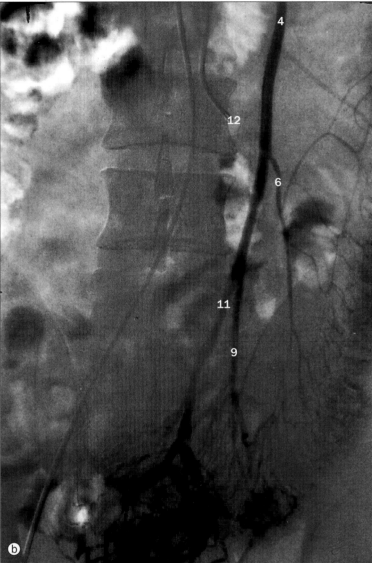

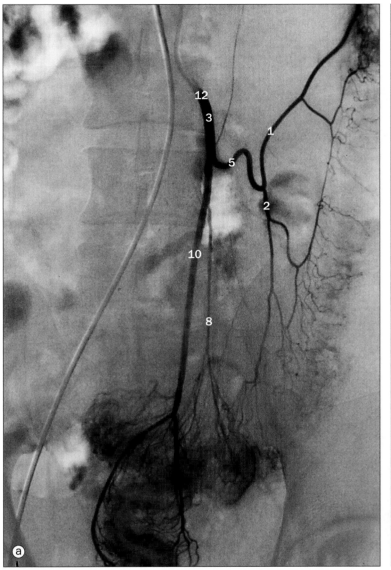

(a) Subtracted inferior mesenteric arteriogram.

(b) Venous phase of subtracted inferior mesenteric arteriogram.

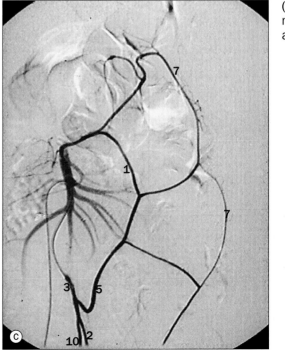

(c) Inferior mesenteric arteriogram.

1 Ascending branch of left colic artery
2 Descending branch of left colic artery
3 Inferior mesenteric artery
4 Inferior mesenteric vein
5 Left colic artery
6 Left colic vein
7 Marginal artery of Drummond
8 Sigmoid arteries
9 Sigmoid vein
10 Superior rectal artery
11 Superior rectal vein
12 Tip of catheter in inferior mesenteric artery

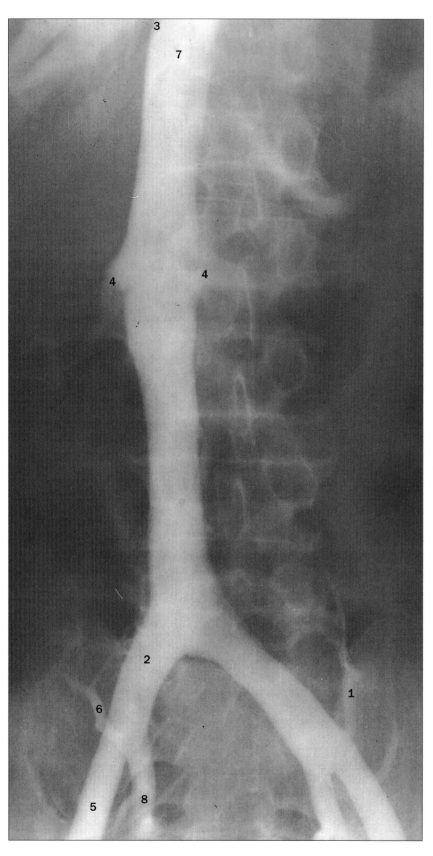

Inferior vena cavogram.

1 Ascending lumbar vein
2 Common iliac vein
3 Entrance of hepatic veins
4 Entrance of renal veins
5 External iliac vein
6 Iliolumbar vein
7 Inferior vena cava
8 Internal iliac vein

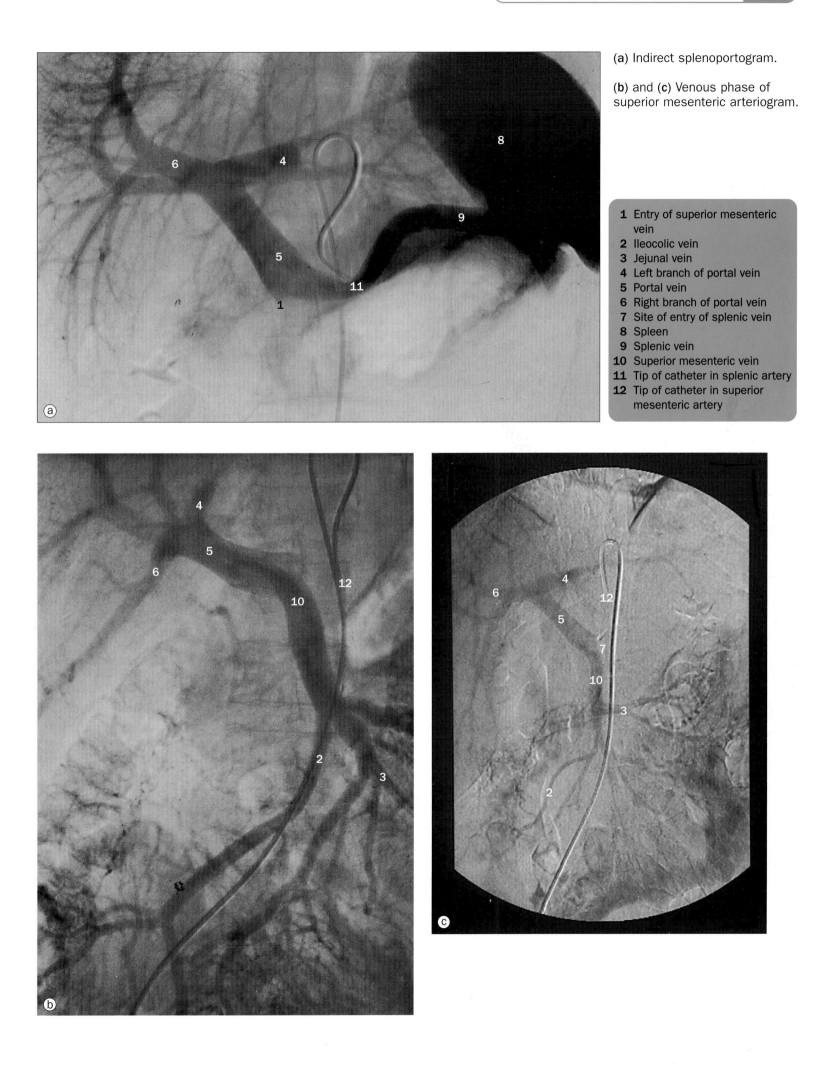

(a) Indirect splenoportogram.

(b) and (c) Venous phase of superior mesenteric arteriogram.

1 Entry of superior mesenteric vein
2 Ileocolic vein
3 Jejunal vein
4 Left branch of portal vein
5 Portal vein
6 Right branch of portal vein
7 Site of entry of splenic vein
8 Spleen
9 Splenic vein
10 Superior mesenteric vein
11 Tip of catheter in splenic artery
12 Tip of catheter in superior mesenteric artery

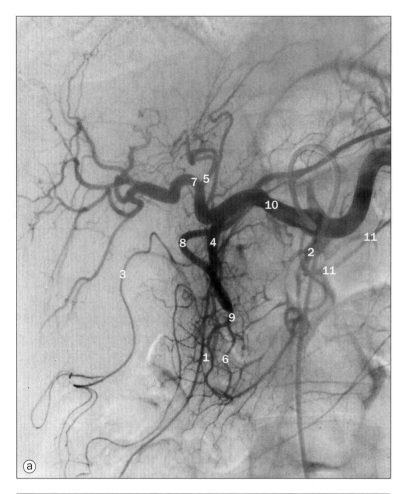

(a) Subtracted hepatic arteriogram.

1 Anterior branch of superior pancreaticoduodenal artery
2 Dorsal pancreatic artery
3 Epiploic arteries
4 Gastroduodenal artery
5 Left branch of hepatic artery
6 Posterior branch of superior pancreaticoduodenal artery
7 Right branch of hepatic artery
8 Right gastro-epiploic artery
9 Superior pancreaticoduodenal artery
10 Tip of catheter in hepatic artery
11 Transverse pancreatic artery

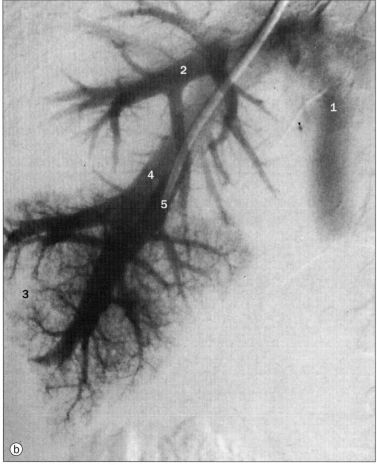

(b) Subtracted hepatic venogram.

1 Inferior vena cava
2 Middle hepatic vein
3 Parenchyma of liver
4 Right hepatic vein
5 Tip of catheter in hepatic vein

(a) Selective gastroduodenal arteriogram.
(b) Subtracted pancreatic arteriogram.

1 Anterior branch of inferior pancreaticoduodenal artery
2 Anterior branch of superior pancreaticoduodenal artery
3 Gastroduodenal artery
4 Left gastro-epiploic artery
5 Posterior branch of inferior pancreaticoduodenal artery
6 Posterior branch of superior pancreaticoduodenal artery
7 Right gastro-epiploic artery
8 Superior mesenteric artery
9 Tip of catheter in dorsal pancreatic artery
10 Transverse pancreatic artery

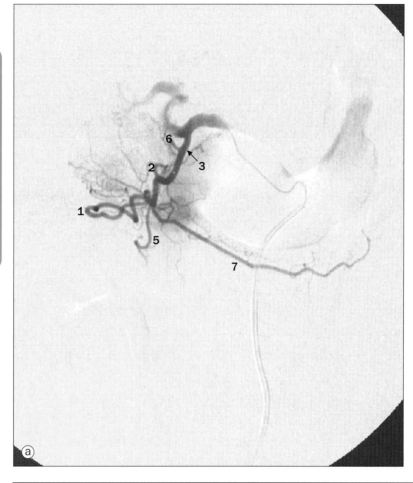

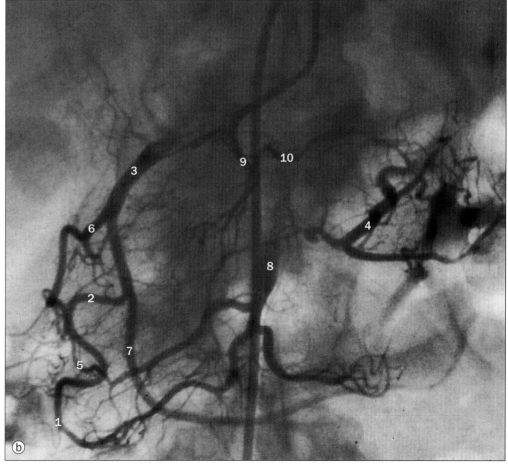

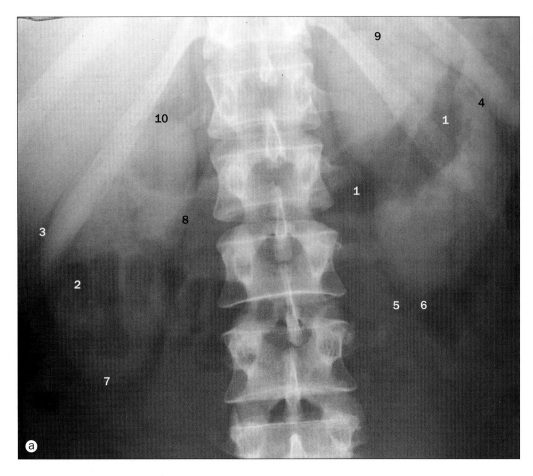

(a) Nephrographic phase of an excretion urogram.

1	Gas in stomach
2	Gas in transverse colon
3	Lateral border of right kidney
4	Lateral margin of left kidney
5	Left psoas muscle
6	Lower pole of left kidney
7	Lower pole of right kidney
8	Right psoas muscle
9	Upper pole of left kidney
10	Upper pole of right kidney

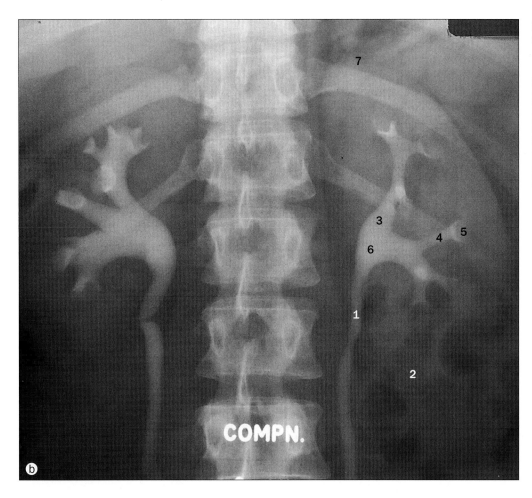

(b) Pyelographic phase of an excretion urogram.

1	Left ureter
2	Lower pole of left kidney
3	Major calyx
4	Minor calyx
5	Renal papilla
6	Renal pelvis
7	Upper pole of left kidney

Intravenous urogram 15 min film.

1 Gas in the ascending colon
2 Gas in the descending colon
3 Gas in the duodenal cap (first part of
   the duodenum)
4 Gas in the ileum
5 Gas in the jejunum
6 Gas in the stomach
7 Left ureter
8 Lower pole of left kidney
9 Major calyx
10 Minor calyx
11 Renal papilla
12 Renal pelvis
13 Tip of the right lobe of the liver
14 Upper pole of left kidney

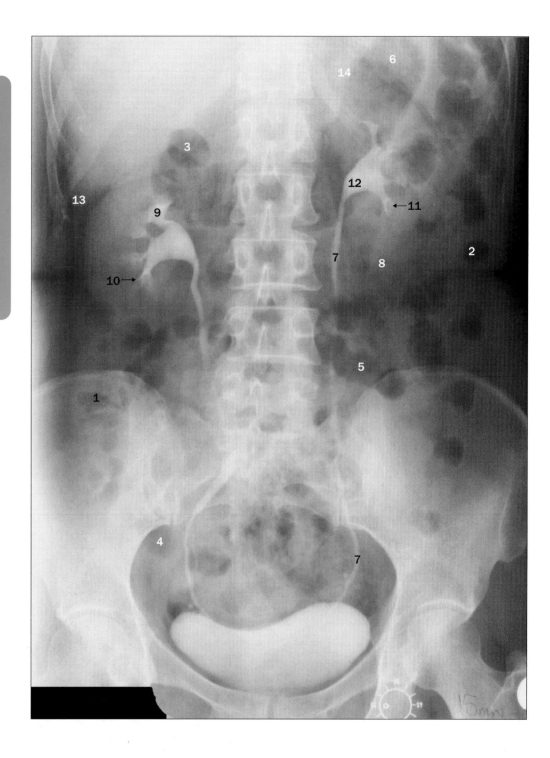

(a) Renal arteriogram.

1 Arcuate arteries
2 Interlobar arteries
3 Lobar arteries
4 Main renal artery
5 Tip of catheter in renal artery

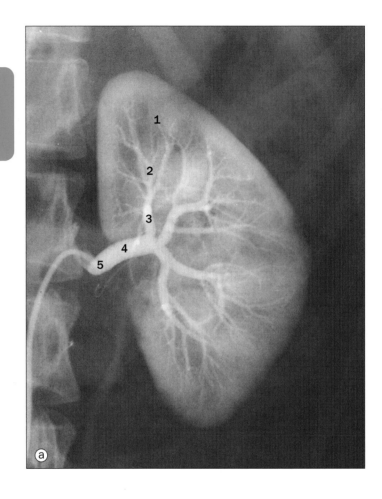

(b) Left renal venogram.

1 Arcuate veins
2 Catheter in left renal artery
3 Catheter in left renal vein
4 Inferior vena cava
5 Interlobar veins
6 Lobar veins
7 Main renal vein

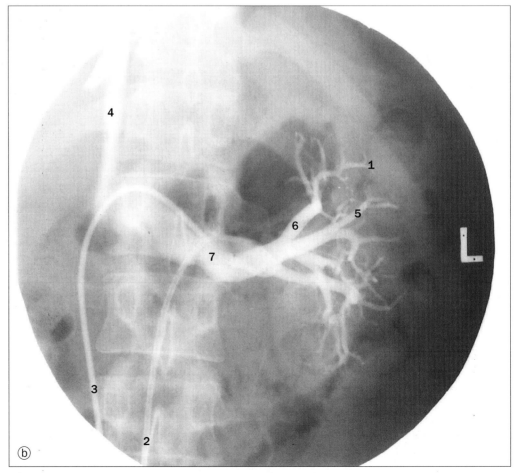

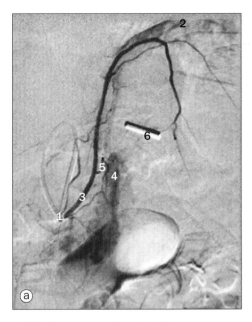

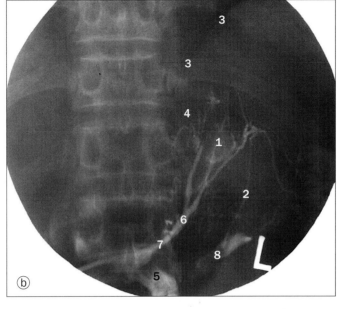

(b) Left suprarenal venogram.

Angiography of the suprarenal glands has been superseded by other imaging techniques. Although there is a wide variation, the arterial supply to the suprarenal glands is from three main arteries: the inferior suprarenal artery, which comes off the renal artery; the middle suprarenal artery, directly off the aorta; and the superior suprarenal artery, arising from the inferior phrenic artery. Suprarenal venous sampling is still performed in some centres as part of the localisation of hormone-secreting tumours.

(a) Left suprarenal arteriogram.

1	Catheter in origin of inferior phrenic artery
2	Diaphragm
3	Inferior phrenic artery
4	Left suprarenal gland
5	Superior suprarenal arteries
6	Tip of nasogastric tube

1	Adenoma in suprarenal gland	5	Left renal vein
2	Capsular veins	6	Left suprarenal vein
3	Diaphragm	7	Tip of catheter in left suprarenal vein
4	Inferior phrenic vein	8	Upper pole calyx

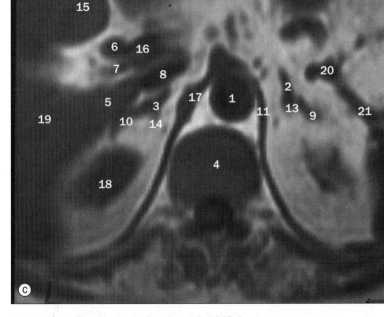

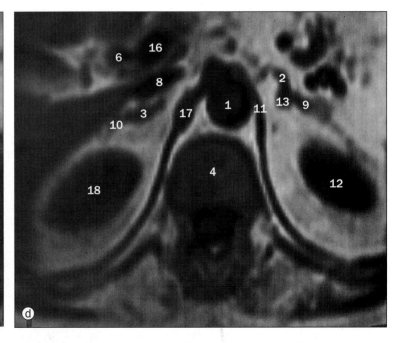

(c) and (d) Suprarenal glands, axial MR images.

1	Aorta	8	Inferior vena cava	15	Medial segment of left lobe of liver
2	Body of left suprarenal gland	9	Lateral limb of left suprarenal gland	16	Portal vein
3	Body of right suprarenal gland	10	Lateral limb of right suprarenal gland	17	Right crus of diaphragm
4	Body of vertebra	11	Left crus of diaphragm	18	Right kidney
5	Caudate lobe of liver	12	Left kidney	19	Right lobe of liver
6	Common bile duct	13	Medial limb of left suprarenal gland	20	Splenic artery
7	Hepatic artery	14	Medial limb of right suprarenal gland	21	Splenic vein

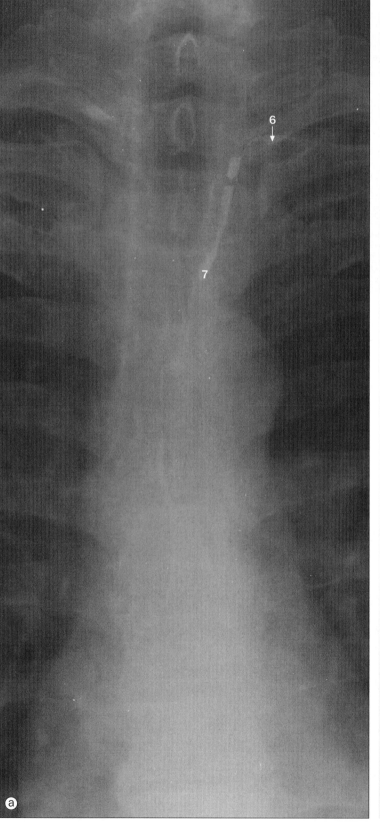

Lymphangiograms, (a) of the thorax and upper abdomen, (b) of the paralumbar region.

1 Ascending lumbar chains
2 Cisterna chyli
3 Efferent inguinal lymphatics
4 External iliac nodes (early filling)
5 Inguinal nodes (early filling)
6 Terminal ampulla
7 Thoracic duct

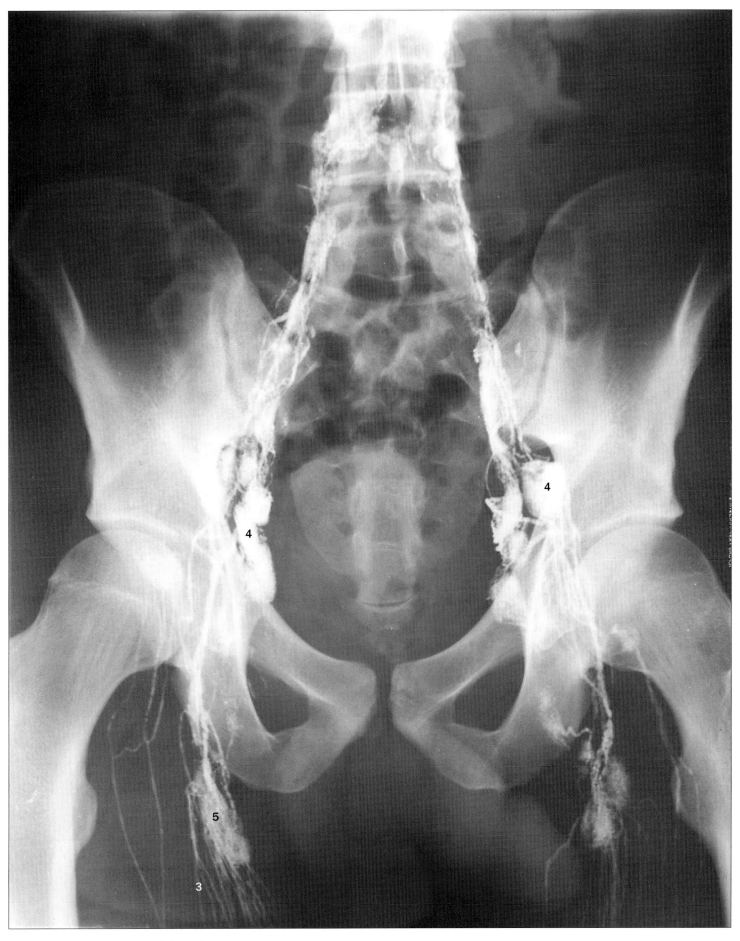

Lymphangiogram of the pelvic region.
See page 152 for key.

6 Pelvis

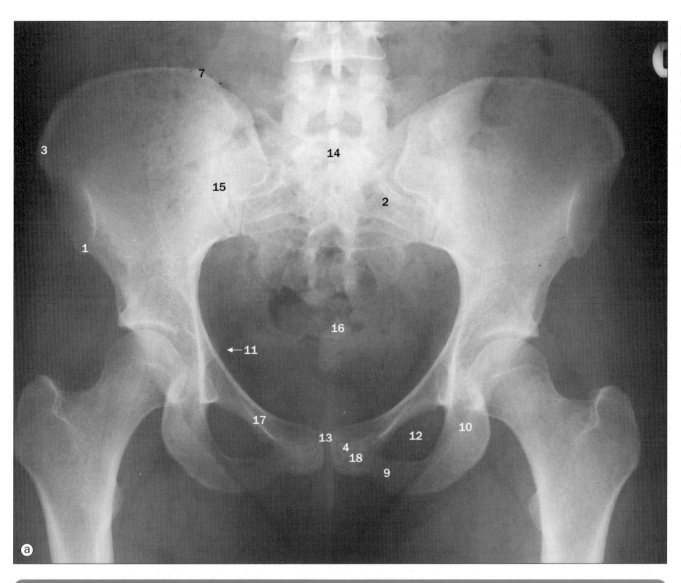

(a) Pelvis and hips of an adult female, anteroposterior projection.
(b) and (c) Pelvis of a 17-year-old male, anteroposterior projections.

1 Anterior inferior iliac spine	**7** Iliac crest	**13** Pubic symphysis
2 Anterior sacral foramen	**8** Ilium	**14** Sacral crest
3 Anterior superior iliac spine	**9** Inferior ramus of pubis	**15** Sacro-iliac joint
4 Body of pubis	**10** Ischial ramus	**16** Segment of coccyx
5 Centre for iliac crest	**11** Ischial spine	**17** Superior ramus of pubis
6 Centre for ischial tuberosity	**12** Obturator foramen	**18** Tubercle of pubis

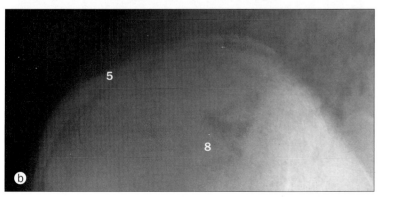

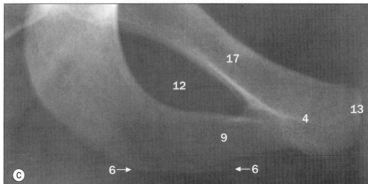

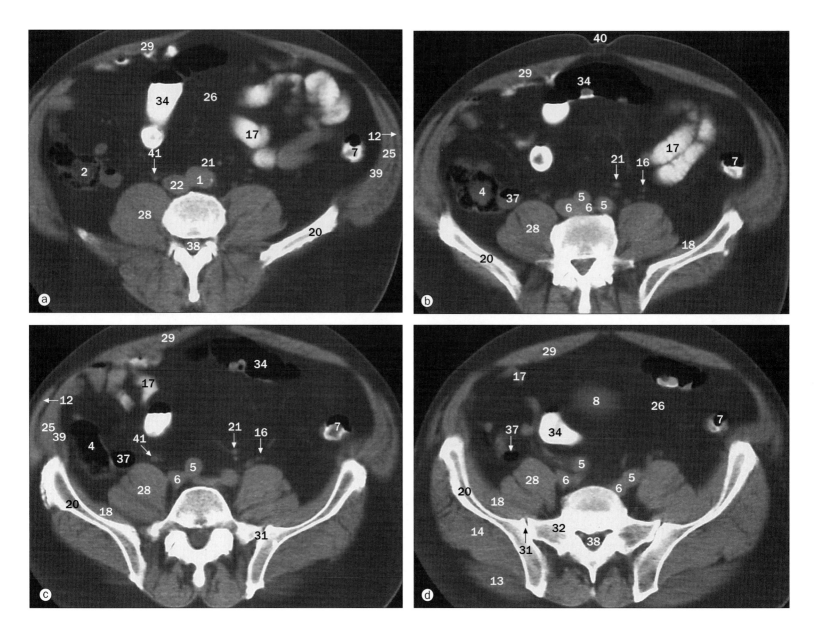

(a)–(h) Male pelvis, axial CT images.

1 Aorta	**11** External iliac vein
2 Ascending colon	**12** External oblique muscle
3 Bladder	**13** Gluteus maximus muscle
4 Caecum	**14** Gluteus medius muscle
5 Common iliac artery	**15** Gluteus minimus muscle
6 Common iliac vein	**16** Gonadal artery and vein
7 Descending colon	**17** Ileal loop
8 Dome of bladder	**18** Iliacus muscle
9 Dorsal sacral foramen	**19** Iliopsoas muscle
10 External iliac artery	**20** Ilium

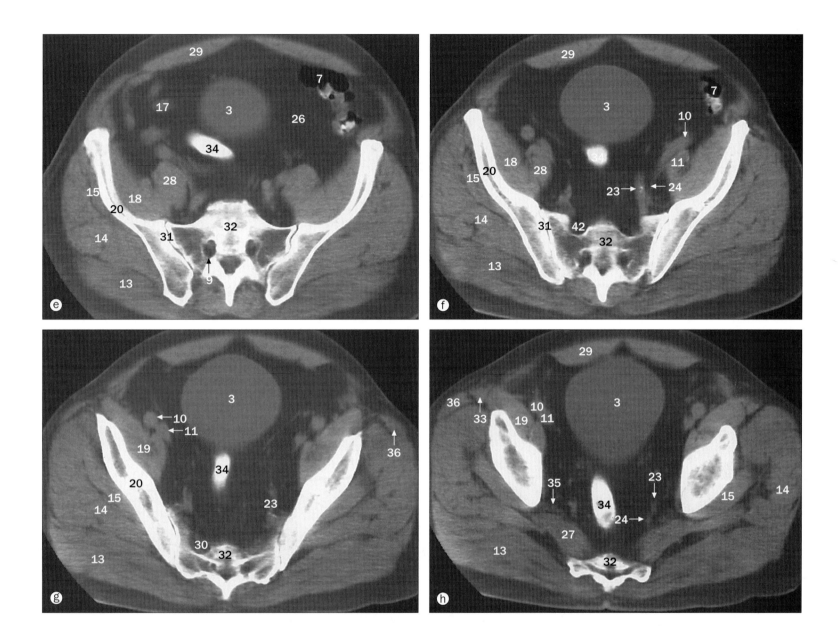

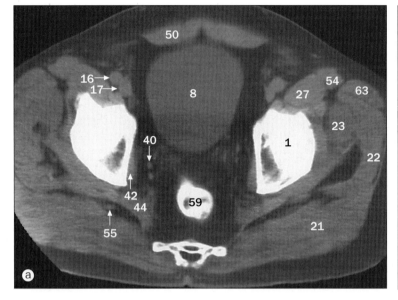
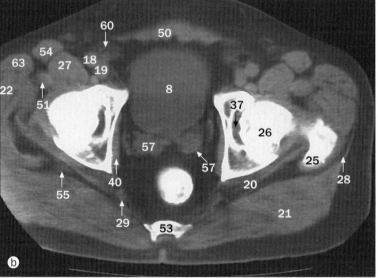
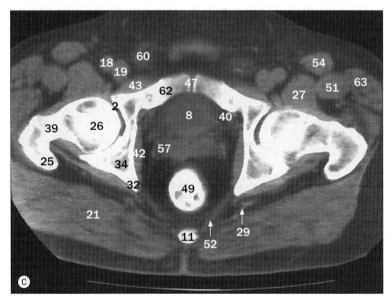

(a)–(i) Male pelvis, axial CT images.

1 Acetabular roof	**23** Gluteus minimus muscle	**45** Profunda femoris artery
2 Acetabulum	**24** Gracilis muscle	**46** Prostate
3 Adductor brevis muscle	**25** Greater trochanter of femur	**47** Pubic symphysis
4 Adductor longus muscle	**26** Head of femur	**48** Quadratus femoris muscle
5 Adductor magnus muscle	**27** Iliopsoas muscle	**49** Rectum
6 Anal canal	**28** Iliotibial tract	**50** Rectus abdominis muscle
7 Biceps femoris muscle	**29** Inferior gluteal artery and vein	**51** Rectus femoris muscle
8 Bladder	**30** Inferior ramus of pubis	**52** Sacrospinous ligament
9 Body of pubis	**31** Internal pudendal artery and vein	**53** Sacrum
10 Bulb of penis	**32** Ischial spine	**54** Sartorius muscle
11 Coccyx	**33** Ischio-anal fossa	**55** Sciatic nerve
12 Corpus cavernosum	**34** Ischium	**56** Semimembranosus muscle
13 Crus of corpus cavernosum	**35** Lesser trochanter of femur	**57** Seminal vesicle
14 Epididymis	**36** Levator ani muscle	**58** Semitendinosus muscle
15 External anal sphincter	**37** Ligament of head of femur	**59** Sigmoid colon
16 External iliac artery	**38** Membranous urethra	**60** Spermatic cord
17 External iliac vein	**39** Neck of femur	**61** Superficial femoral artery
18 Femoral artery	**40** Obturator artery and vein	**62** Superior ramus of pubis
19 Femoral vein	**41** Obturator externus muscle	**63** Tensor fasciae latae muscle
20 Gemellus muscle	**42** Obturator internus muscle	**64** Testis
21 Gluteus maximus muscle	**43** Pectineus muscle	**65** Vastus intermedius muscle
22 Gluteus medius muscle	**44** Piriformis muscle	**66** Vastus lateralis muscle

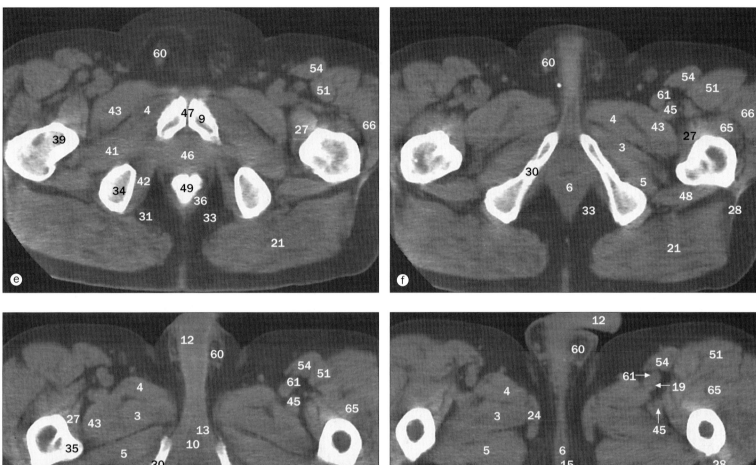

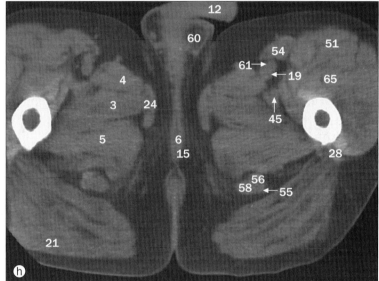

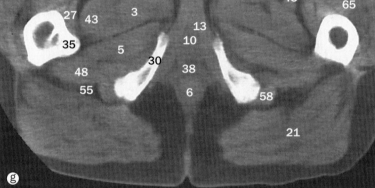

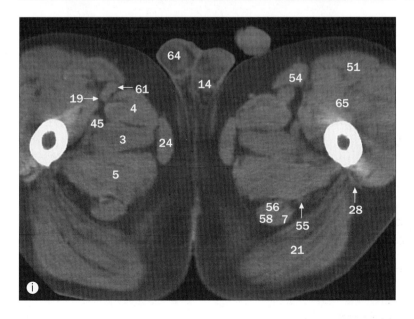

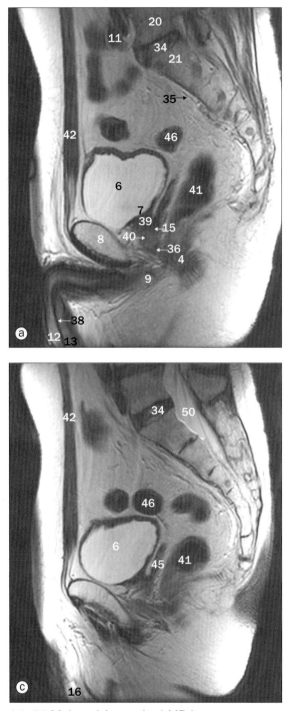

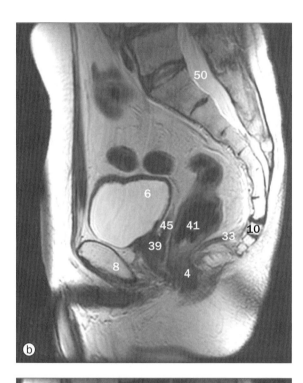

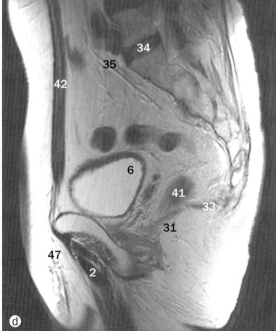

(a)–(h) Male pelvis, sagittal MR images.

1 Adductor brevis muscle	**13** Corpus spongiosum
2 Adductor longus muscle	**14** Descending colon
3 Adductor magnus muscle	**15** Ejaculatory duct
4 Anal canal	**16** Epididymis
5 Aorta	**17** External iliac artery
6 Bladder	**18** External iliac vein
7 Bladder neck	**19** Femoral artery
8 Body of pubis	**20** Fifth lumbar vertebra
9 Bulb of penis	**21** First sacral segment
10 Coccyx	**22** Gemellus muscle
11 Common iliac vein	**23** Gluteus maximus muscle
12 Corpus cavernosum	**24** Iliacus muscle

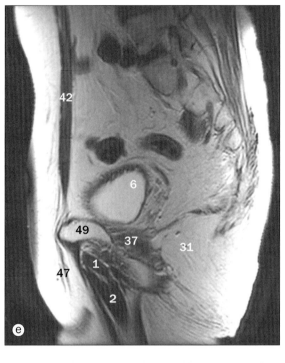

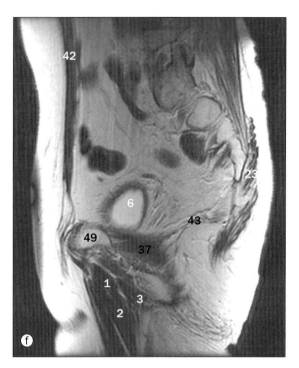

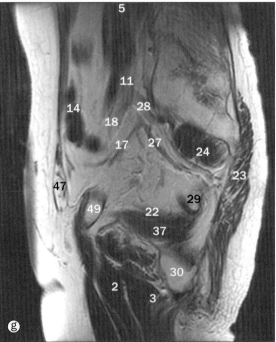

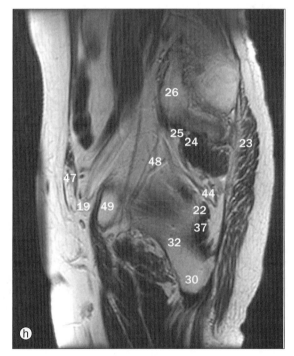

25 Iliopsoas muscle	**38** Penile urethra
26 Ilium	**39** Prostate
27 Internal iliac artery	**40** Prostatic urethra
28 Internal iliac vein	**41** Rectum
29 Ischial spine	**42** Rectus abdominis muscle
30 Ischial tuberosity	**43** Sacrospinous ligament
31 Ischio-anal fossa	**44** Sciatic nerve
32 Ischium	**45** Seminal vesicle
33 Levator ani muscle	**46** Sigmoid colon
34 Lumbosacral disc	**47** Spermatic cord
35 Median sacral artery	**48** Superior gluteal artery and vein
36 Membranous urethra	**49** Superior ramus of pubis
37 Obturator internus muscle	**50** Thecal sac

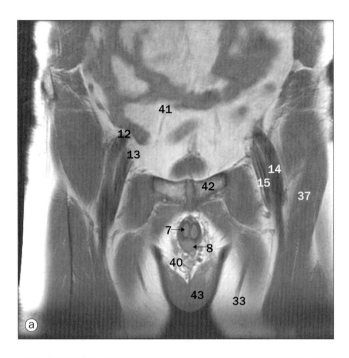

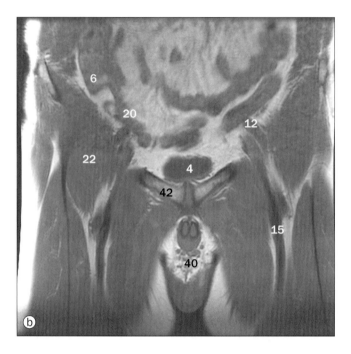

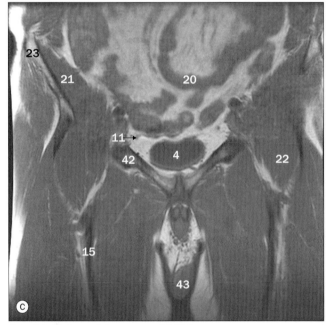

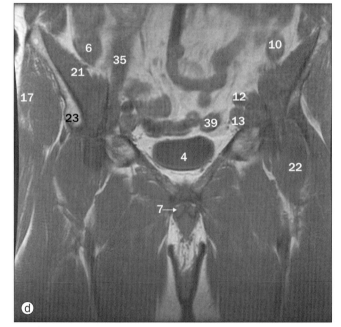

(a)–(h) Male pelvis, coronal MR images.

1 Acetabular roof	**12** External iliac artery
2 Acetabulum	**13** External iliac vein
3 Anal canal	**14** Femoral artery
4 Bladder	**15** Femoral vein
5 Bulb of penis	**16** Fifth lumbar vertebra
6 Caecum	**17** Gluteus medius muscle
7 Corpus cavernosum	**18** Gluteus minimus muscle
8 Corpus spongiosum	**19** Head of femur
9 Crus of corpus cavernosum	**20** Ileal loop
10 Descending colon	**21** Iliacus muscle
11 Ductus deferens (vas deferens)	**22** Iliopsoas muscle

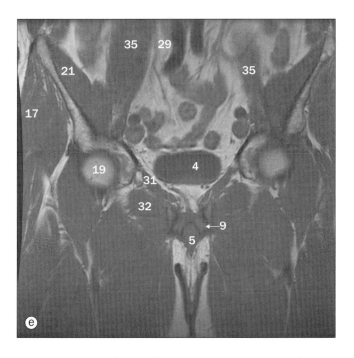

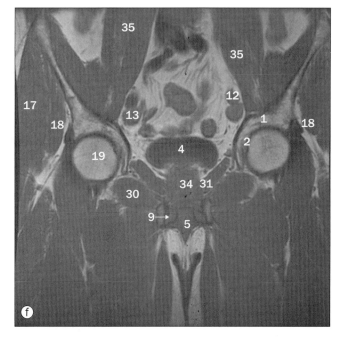

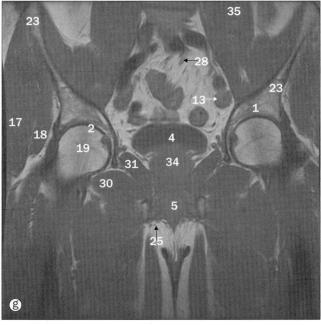

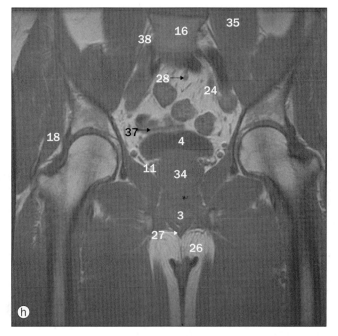

23 Ilium	**34** Prostate
24 Inferior gluteal artery and vein	**35** Psoas muscle
25 Internal pudendal artery and vein	**36** Rectum
26 Ischio-anal fossa	**37** Sartorius muscle
27 Levator ani muscle	**38** Sciatic nerve root
28 Median sacral artery	**39** Sigmoid colon
29 Mesenteric fat	**40** Spermatic cord
30 Obturator externus muscle	**41** Superficial epigastric artery
31 Obturator internus muscle	**42** Superior ramus of pubis
32 Pectineus muscle	**43** Testis
33 Profunda femoris artery	

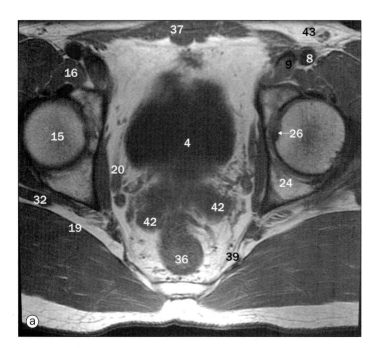

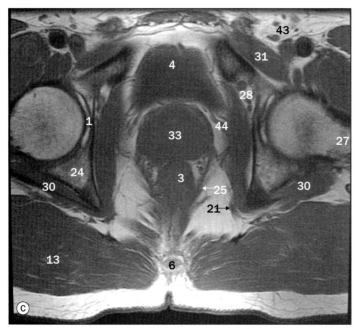

(a)–(d) Male pelvis, axial MR images.

1 Acetabulum	12 Femoral vein
2 Adductor longus muscle	13 Gluteus maximus muscle
3 Anal canal	14 Greater trochanter of femur
4 Bladder	15 Head of femur
5 Body of pubis	16 Iliopsoas muscle
6 Coccyx	17 Inferior gluteal artery and vein
7 Corpus cavernosum	18 Inferior pubic ramus
8 External iliac artery	19 Internal iliac artery
9 External iliac vein	20 Internal iliac vein
10 Femoral artery	21 Internal pudendal artery and vein
11 Femoral nerve	22 Ischial tuberosity

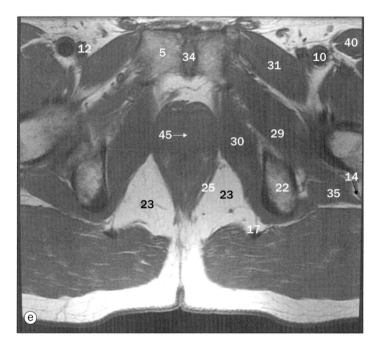

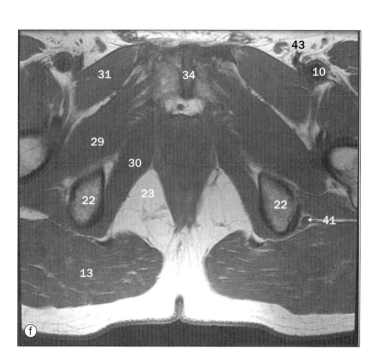

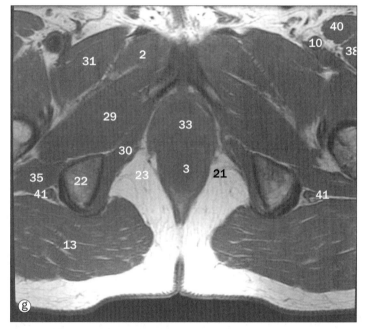

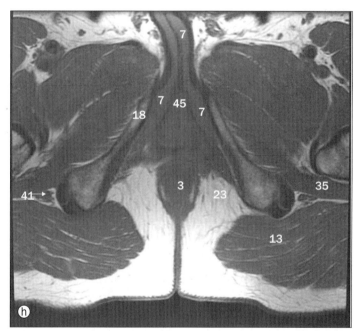

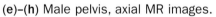

(e)–(h) Male pelvis, axial MR images.

23	Ischio-anal fossa	35	Quadratus femoris muscle
24	Ischium	36	Rectum
25	Levator ani muscle	37	Rectus abdominis muscle
26	Ligament of head of femur	38	Rectus femoris muscle
27	Neck of femur	39	Sacrospinous ligament
28	Obturator artery and vein	40	Sartorius muscle
29	Obturator externus muscle	41	Sciatic nerve
30	Obturator internus muscle	42	Seminal vesicle
31	Pectineus muscle	43	Spermatic cord
32	Piriformis muscle	44	Ureter
33	Prostate	45	Urethra
34	Pubic symphysis		

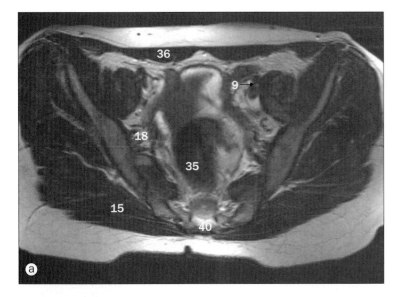

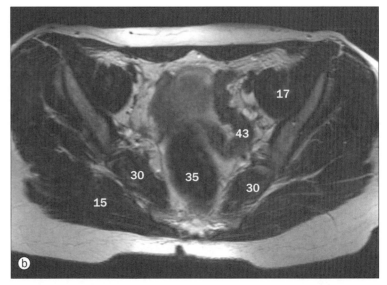

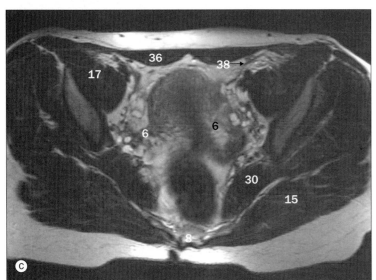

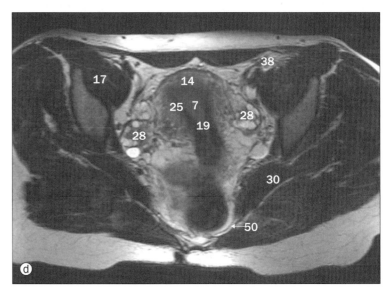

(a)–(l) Female pelvis, axial MR images.

1 Acetabular roof	**14** Fundus of uterus
2 Acetabulum	**15** Gluteus maximus muscle
3 Anal canal	**16** Head of femur
4 Bladder	**17** Iliopsoas muscle
5 Body of pubis	**18** Internal iliac artery and vein
6 Broad ligament	**19** Internal os of cervix
7 Cavity of uterus	**20** Internal pudendal artery and vein
8 Coccyx	**21** Ischial spine
9 External iliac artery and vein	**22** Ischio-anal fossa
10 External os of cervix	**23** Ischium
11 Femoral artery	**24** Levator ani muscle
12 Femoral nerve	**25** Myometrium of uterus
13 Femoral vein	**26** Obturator externus muscle

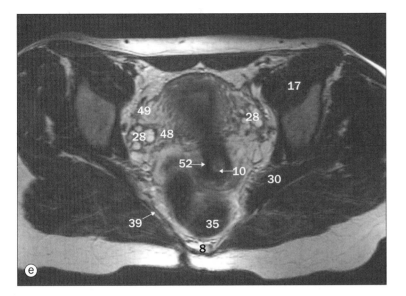

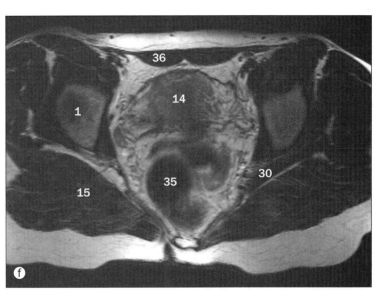

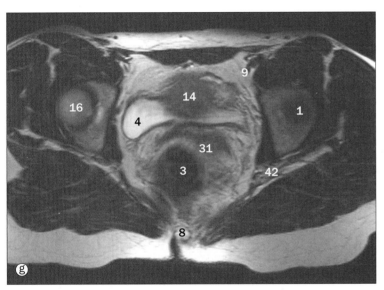

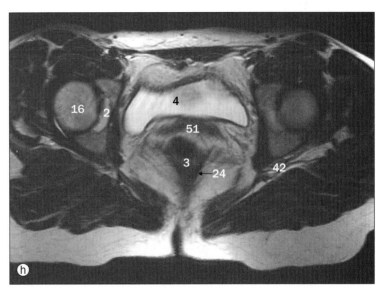

(e)–(h) Female pelvis, axial MR images.

27 Obturator internus muscle	40 Sacrum
28 Ovary	41 Sartorius muscle
29 Pectineus muscle	42 Sciatic nerve
30 Piriformis muscle	43 Sigmoid colon
31 Posterior fornix of vagina	44 Superficial femoral artery
32 Profunda femoris artery	45 Superficial femoral vein
33 Pubic symphysis	46 Tensor fasciae latae muscle
34 Quadratus femoris muscle	47 Urethra
35 Rectum	48 Uterine artery
36 Rectus abdominis muscle	49 Uterine tube
37 Rectus femoris muscle	50 Uterosacral ligament
38 Round ligament	51 Vagina
39 Sacrospinous ligament	52 Wall of cervix

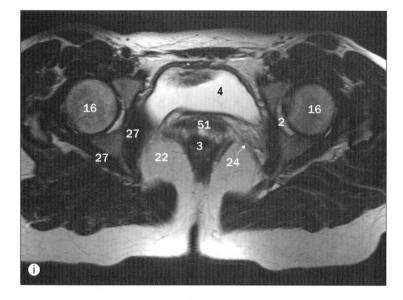

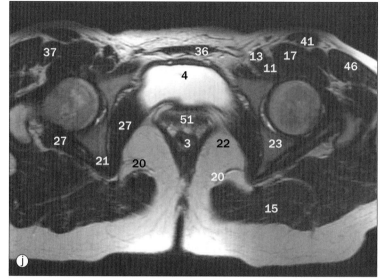

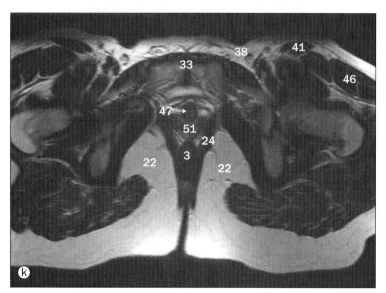

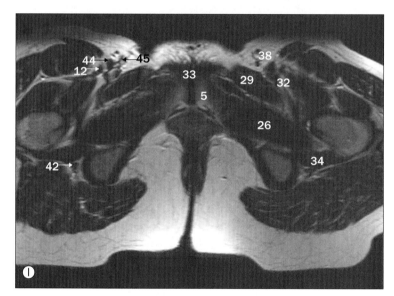

(i)–(l) Female pelvis, axial MR images.

1 Acetabular roof	**19** Internal os of cervix	**37** Rectus femoris muscle
2 Acetabulum	**20** Internal pudendal artery and vein	**38** Round ligament
3 Anal canal	**21** Ischial spine	**39** Sacrospinous ligament
4 Bladder	**22** Ischio-anal fossa	**40** Sacrum
5 Body of pubis	**23** Ischium	**41** Sartorius muscle
6 Broad ligament	**24** Levator ani muscle	**42** Sciatic nerve
7 Cavity of uterus	**25** Myometrium of uterus	**43** Sigmoid colon
8 Coccyx	**26** Obturator externus muscle	**44** Superficial femoral artery
9 External iliac artery and vein	**27** Obturator internus muscle	**45** Superficial femoral vein
10 External os of cervix	**28** Ovary	**46** Tensor fasciae latae muscle
11 Femoral artery	**29** Pectineus muscle	**47** Urethra
12 Femoral nerve	**30** Piriformis muscle	**48** Uterine artery
13 Femoral vein	**31** Posterior fornix of vagina	**49** Uterine tube
14 Fundus of uterus	**32** Profunda femoris artery	**50** Uterosacral ligament
15 Gluteus maximus muscle	**33** Pubic symphysis	**51** Vagina
16 Head of femur	**34** Quadratus femoris muscle	**52** Wall of cervix
17 Iliopsoas muscle	**35** Rectum	
18 Internal iliac artery and vein	**36** Rectus abdominis muscle	

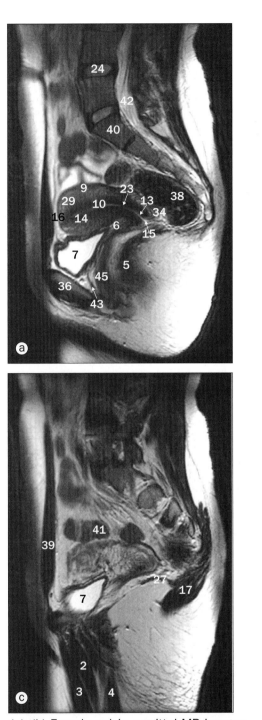

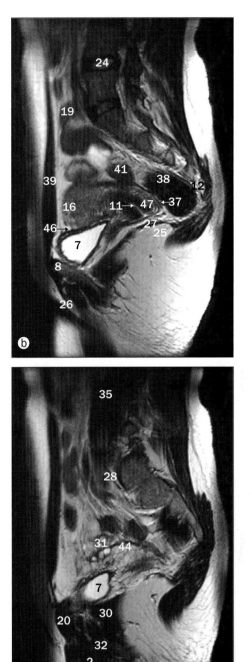

(a)–(h) Female pelvis, sagittal MR images.

1 Acetabular fossa	**13** Endocervical canal of cervix	**25** Ischio-anal fossa	**37** Recto-uterine pouch
2 Adductor brevis muscle	**14** Endometrium	**26** Labium majus	**38** Rectum
3 Adductor longus muscle	**15** External os of cervix	**27** Levator ani muscle	**39** Rectus abdominis muscle
4 Adductor magnus muscle	**16** Fundus of uterus	**28** Median sacral artery	**40** Sacrum
5 Anal canal	**17** Gluteus maximus muscle	**29** Myometrium of uterus	**41** Sigmoid colon
6 Anterior fornix of vagina	**18** Head of femur	**30** Obturator internus muscle	**42** Thecal sac
7 Bladder	**19** Ileum	**31** Ovary	**43** Urethra
8 Body of pubis	**20** Iliacus muscle	**32** Pectineus muscle	**44** Uterine tube
9 Body of uterus	**21** Ilium	**33** Piriformis muscle	**45** Vagina
10 Cavity of uterus	**22** Internal iliac artery and vein	**34** Posterior fornix of vagina	**46** Vesico-uterine pouch
11 Cervical canal	**23** Internal os of cervix	**35** Psoas muscle	**47** Wall of cervix
12 Coccyx	**24** Intervertebral disc	**36** Pubic symphysis	

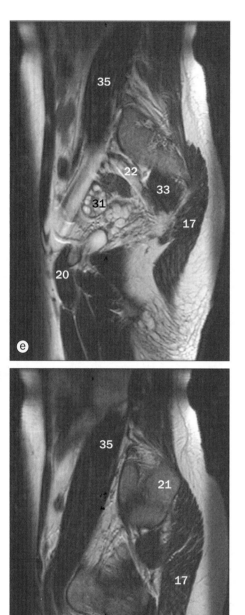

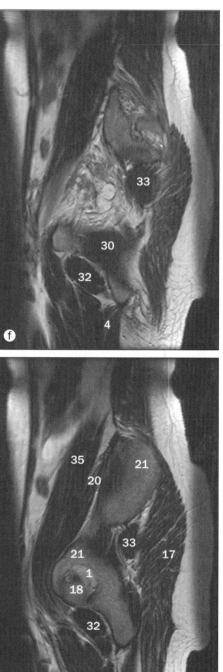

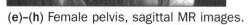

(e)–(h) Female pelvis, sagittal MR images.

1 Acetabular fossa	**13** Endocervical canal of cervix	**25** Ischio-anal fossa	**37** Recto-uterine pouch
2 Adductor brevis muscle	**14** Endometrium	**26** Labium majus	**38** Rectum
3 Adductor longus muscle	**15** External os of cervix	**27** Levator ani muscle	**39** Rectus abdominis muscle
4 Adductor magnus muscle	**16** Fundus of uterus	**28** Median sacral artery	**40** Sacrum
5 Anal canal	**17** Gluteus maximus muscle	**29** Myometrium of uterus	**41** Sigmoid colon
6 Anterior fornix of vagina	**18** Head of femur	**30** Obturator internus muscle	**42** Thecal sac
7 Bladder	**19** Ileum	**31** Ovary	**43** Urethra
8 Body of pubis	**20** Iliacus muscle	**32** Pectineus muscle	**44** Uterine tube
9 Body of uterus	**21** Ilium	**33** Piriformis muscle	**45** Vagina
10 Cavity of uterus	**22** Internal iliac artery and vein	**34** Posterior fornix of vagina	**46** Vesico-uterine pouch
11 Cervical canal	**23** Internal os of cervix	**35** Psoas muscle	**47** Wall of cervix
12 Coccyx	**24** Intervertebral disc	**36** Pubic symphysis	

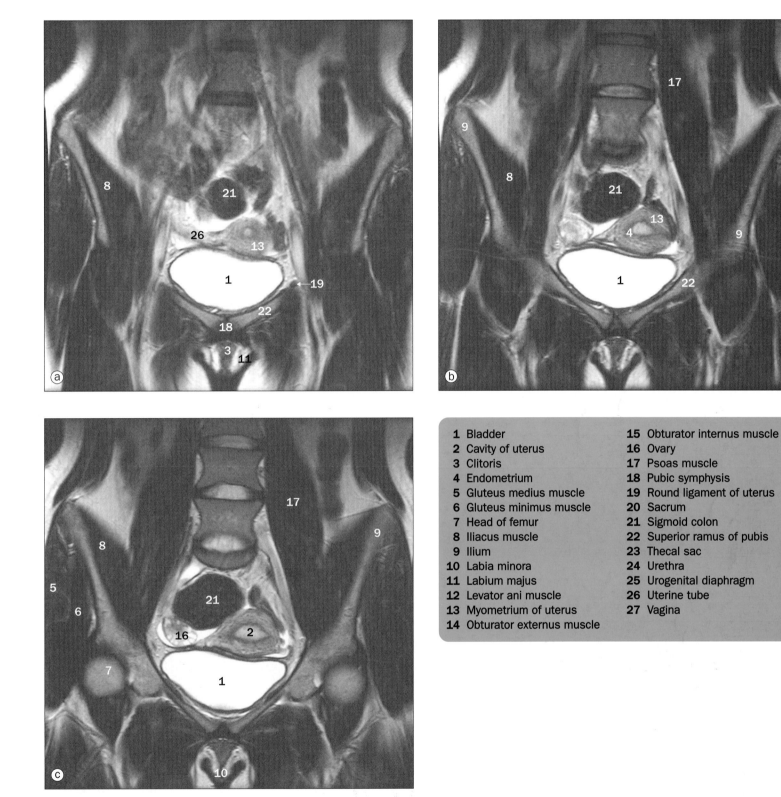

1 Bladder	**15** Obturator internus muscle
2 Cavity of uterus	**16** Ovary
3 Clitoris	**17** Psoas muscle
4 Endometrium	**18** Pubic symphysis
5 Gluteus medius muscle	**19** Round ligament of uterus
6 Gluteus minimus muscle	**20** Sacrum
7 Head of femur	**21** Sigmoid colon
8 Iliacus muscle	**22** Superior ramus of pubis
9 Ilium	**23** Thecal sac
10 Labia minora	**24** Urethra
11 Labium majus	**25** Urogenital diaphragm
12 Levator ani muscle	**26** Uterine tube
13 Myometrium of uterus	**27** Vagina
14 Obturator externus muscle	

(a)–(c) Female pelvis, coronal MR images.

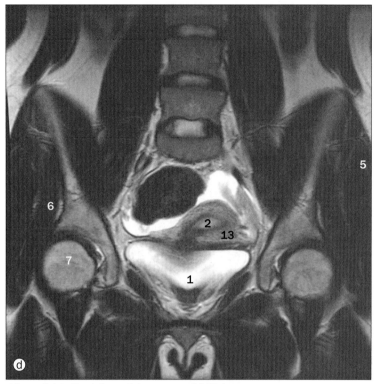 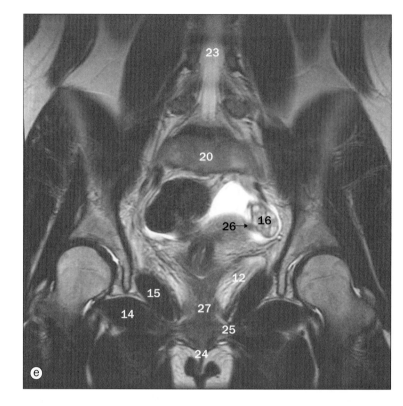

(d) and (e) Female pelvis, coronal MR images.

1	Bladder	**15**	Obturator internus muscle
2	Cavity of uterus	**16**	Ovary
3	Clitoris	**17**	Psoas muscle
4	Endometrium	**18**	Pubic symphysis
5	Gluteus medius muscle	**19**	Round ligament of uterus
6	Gluteus minimus muscle	**20**	Sacrum
7	Head of femur	**21**	Sigmoid colon
8	Iliacus muscle	**22**	Superior ramus of pubis
9	Ilium	**23**	Thecal sac
10	Labia minora	**24**	Urethra
11	Labium majus	**25**	Urogenital diaphragm
12	Levator ani muscle	**26**	Uterine tube
13	Myometrium of uterus	**27**	Vagina
14	Obturator externus muscle		

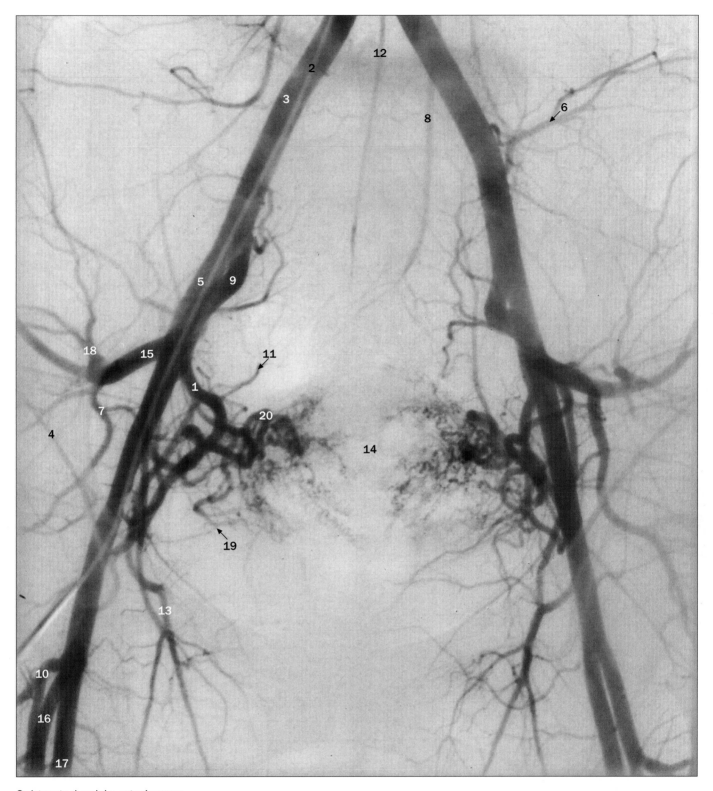

Subtracted pelvic arteriogram.

This anteroposterior film of the pelvis demonstrates both the internal and the external iliac arteries and their branches. Many of the vessels are superimposed: to see them more clearly oblique projections could be obtained. The contrast medium injected into the arteries is excreted by the kidneys, and a full bladder may obscure the branches. Selective catheterisation of the internal and external iliac arteries using a preshaped catheter gives better detail without superimposition of the vessels.

1 Anterior trunk of internal iliac artery	10 Lateral circumflex femoral artery
2 Catheter introduced into distal abdominal aorta via right femoral artery	11 Lateral sacral artery
	12 Median sacral artery
3 Common iliac artery	13 Obturator artery
4 Deep circumflex iliac artery	14 Position of uterus
5 External iliac artery	15 Posterior trunk of internal iliac artery
6 Iliolumbar artery	16 Profunda femoris artery
7 Inferior gluteal artery	17 Superficial femoral artery
8 Inferior mesenteric artery	18 Superior gluteal artery
9 Internal iliac artery	19 Superior vesical artery
	20 Uterine artery

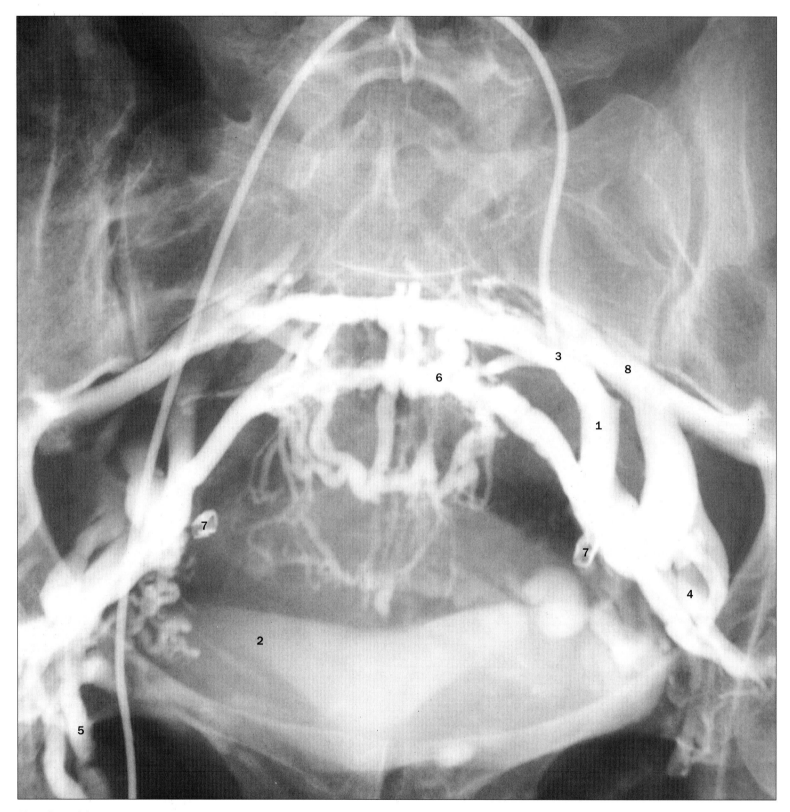

Female pelvic venogram.

1 Anterior division of internal iliac vein
2 Bladder containing contrast medium
3 Catheter introduced via right femoral vein, with tip in left internal iliac vein
4 Inferior gluteal veins
5 Obturator veins
6 Sacral plexus of veins
7 Sterilisation clips
8 Superior gluteal veins

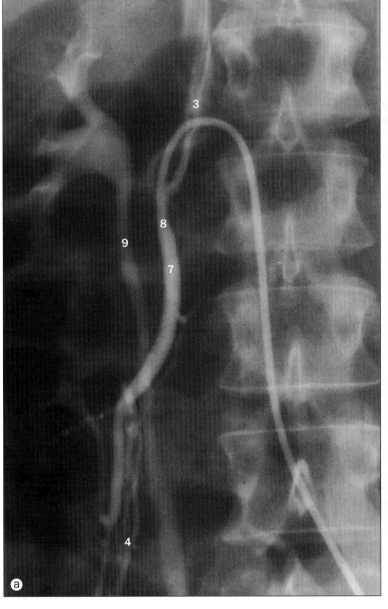

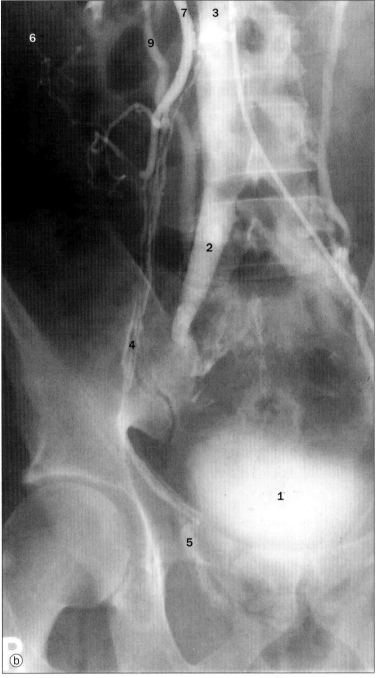

(a) and (b) Right testicular venograms.

The gonadal veins drain into one or two main veins via a venous plexus. On the left, the main vein drains into the left renal vein. It may occasionally communicate with the inferior mesenteric vein and drain into the portal venous system. On the right, the main vein usually drains into the inferior vena cava directly (as in the case illustrated), but it can drain into the right renal vein.

1 Bladder
2 Common iliac veins
3 Inferior vena cava
4 Pampiniform plexus of veins
5 Pampiniform plexus of veins (undescended testis in inguinal canal)
6 Renal capsular veins
7 Right testicular vein
8 Tip of catheter in right testicular vein, introduced via left femoral vein
9 Ureter

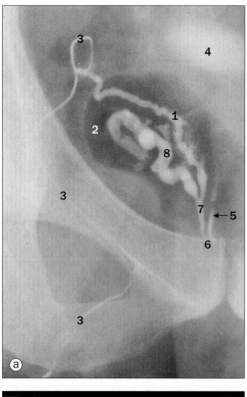

(a) Seminal vesiculogram.

1 Ampulla of ductus deferens
2 Colonic gas
3 Ductus deferens (vas deferens)
4 Full urinary bladder
5 Left ejaculatory duct
6 Position of seminal colliculus (verumontanum)
7 Right ejaculatory duct
8 Seminal vesicle

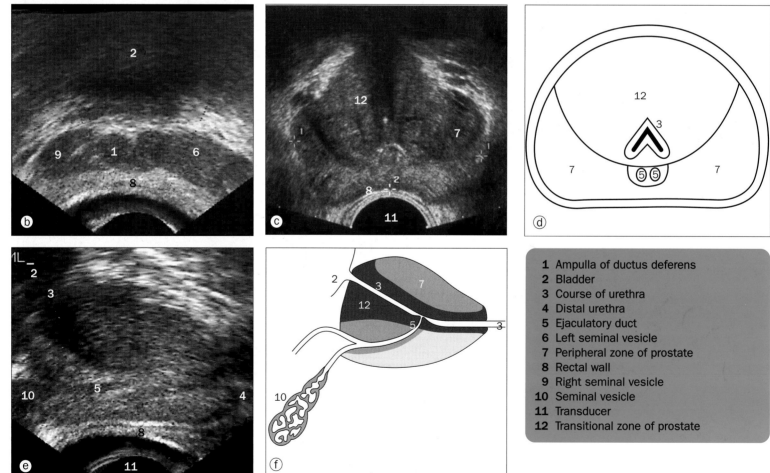

1 Ampulla of ductus deferens
2 Bladder
3 Course of urethra
4 Distal urethra
5 Ejaculatory duct
6 Left seminal vesicle
7 Peripheral zone of prostate
8 Rectal wall
9 Right seminal vesicle
10 Seminal vesicle
11 Transducer
12 Transitional zone of prostate

Rectal ultrasound of the prostate: (b) axial scan through bladder base, (c) axial scan through mid prostate, (d) line drawing of axial scan prostate, (e) sagittal midline scan, (f) line drawing of midline sagittal scan.

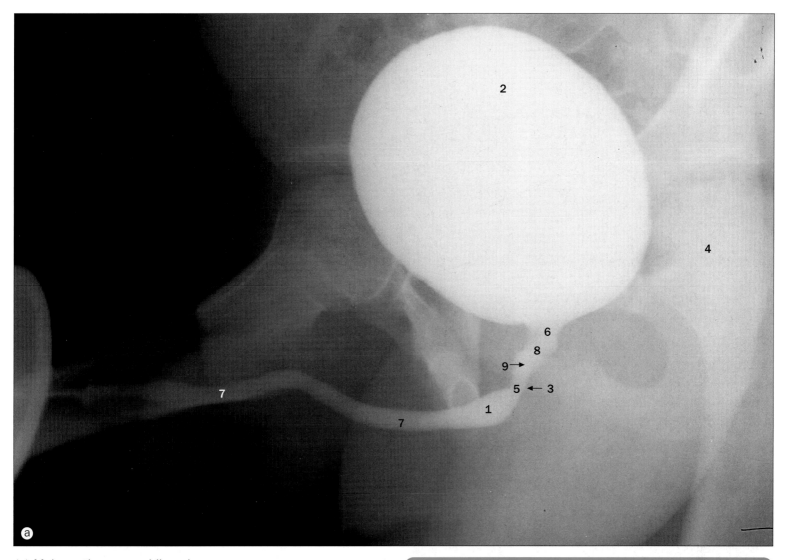

(a) Male urethrogram, oblique image.
(b) Penile arteriogram.
(c) Cavernosogram.

1 Bulbous urethra	**6** Neck of urinary bladder
2 Contrast in urinary bladder	**7** Penile urethra
3 External sphincter	**8** Prostatic urethra
(sphincter urethrae)	**9** Seminal colliculus
4 Head of femur	(verumontanum)
5 Membranous urethra	

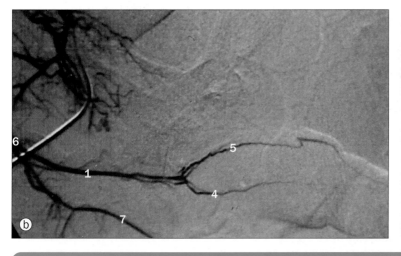

1 Artery of the penis	**5** Dorsal artery of the penis
2 Corpus cavernosum	**6** Internal pudendal artery
3 Crus of corpus cavernosum	**7** Perineal artery
4 Deep artery of the penis	

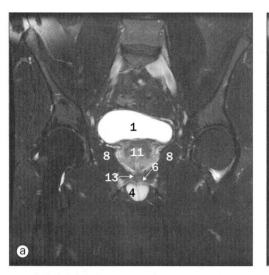

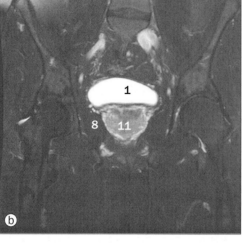

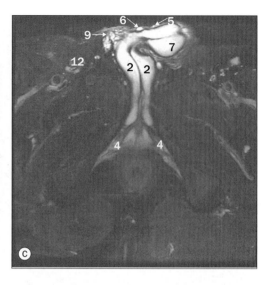

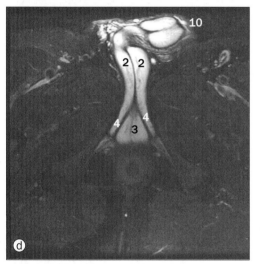

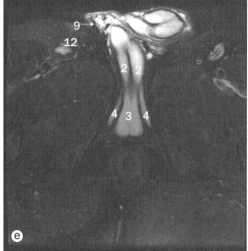

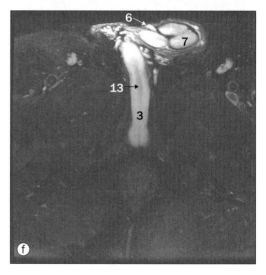

MR images, (a)–(b) coronal, (c)–(f) axial

 1 Bladder
 2 Corpus cavernosum
 3 Corpus spongiosum
 4 Crus of corpus cavernosum
 5 Dorsal artery of penis
 6 Dorsal vein of penis
 7 Glans of penis
 8 Levator ani muscle
 9 Pampiniform plexus of veins
10 Penis
11 Prostate
12 Spermatic cord
13 Urethra

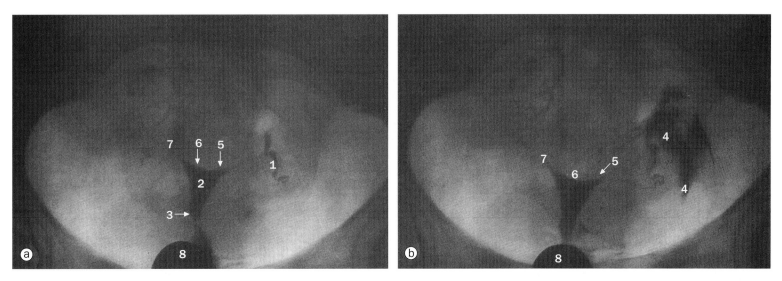

Hysterosalpingograms, (a) immediately after injection, (b) some minutes after injection.

1 Ampulla of uterine tube
2 Body of uterus
3 Cervix of uterus
4 Contrast spillage into peritoneal cavity
5 Cornu of uterus
6 Fundus of uterus
7 Isthmus of uterine tube
8 Speculum in vagina

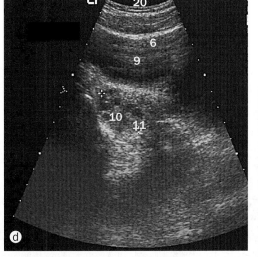

(c) and (d) transvaginal ultrasound of the uterus.
(e) and (f) sagittal MR images, female pelvis.

1 Anal canal
2 Bladder
3 Cavity of uterus
4 Cervix of uterus
5 Coccyx
6 Endometrium
7 Fundus of uterus
8 Labium majus
9 Myometrium of uterus
10 Ovarian follicle
11 Ovary
12 Pubic symphysis
13 Recto-uterine pouch
14 Rectum
15 Round ligament of uterus
16 Sacrum
17 Sigmoid colon
18 Thecal sac
19 Urethra
20 Vagina
21 Vesico-uterine pouch
22 Wall of cervix

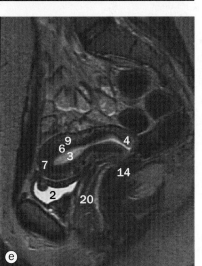

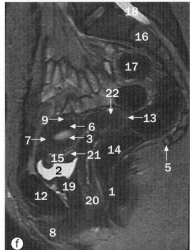

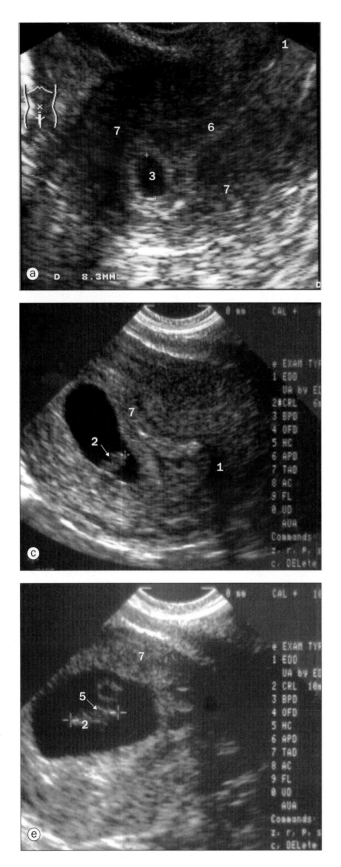
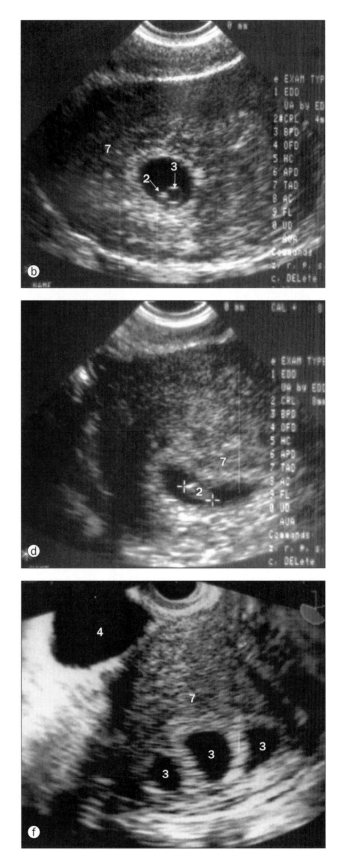

(a) Gestational sac of 8 mms = 5 weeks + 3 days gestational age, (b) CRL (Crown Rump Length) = 4 mms = 6 weeks gestational age, (c) CRL = 6 mms = 6 weeks + 3 days gestational age, (d) CRL = 8 mms = 6 weeks + 5 days gestational age, (e) CRL = 10 mms = 7 weeks + 2 days gestational age, (f) Triplets–3 separate gestational sacs.

1 Cervix	3 Gestation sac	5 Position of fetal heart	7 Uterus
2 Fetus	4 Maternal bladder	6 Uterine cavity	

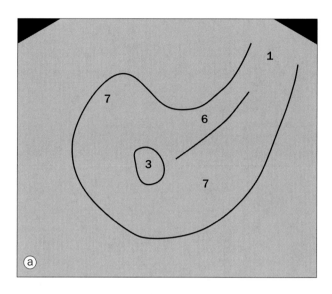

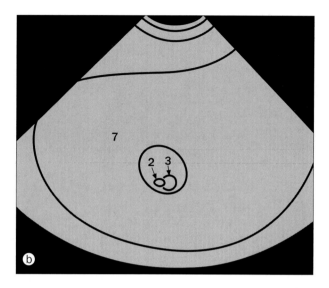

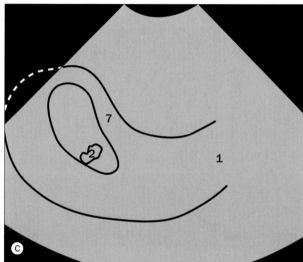

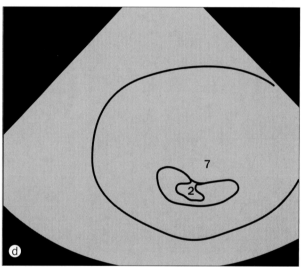

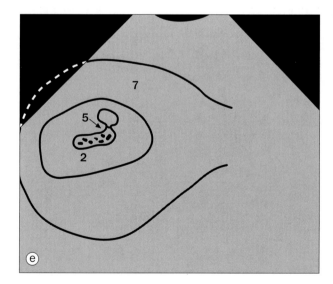

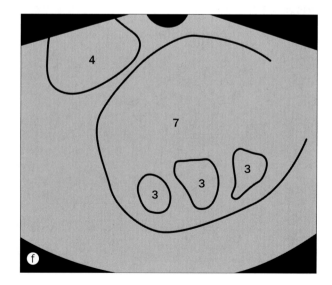

(a)–(f) Line diagrams of ultrasound images opposite.

1 Cervix	3 Gestation sac	5 Position of fetal heart	7 Uterus
2 Fetus	4 Maternal bladder	6 Uterine cavity	

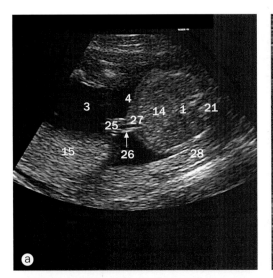

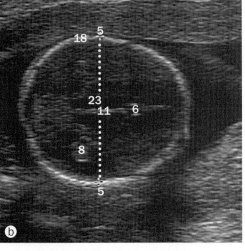

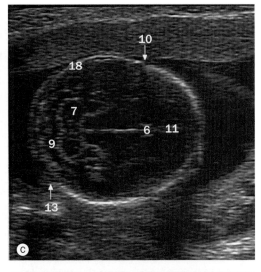

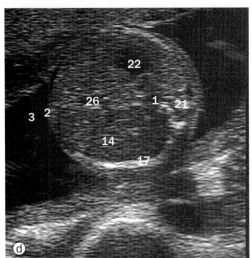

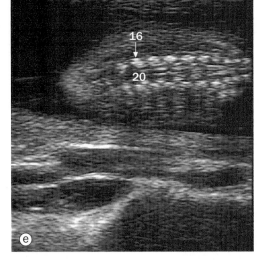

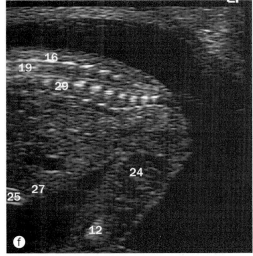

Fetal ultrasound, second trimester:
(a) cord insertion, (b) and (c) skull,
(d) abdomen, (e) and (f) spine.

1 Abdominal aorta	**15** Placenta
2 Abdominal circumference measurement	**16** Posterior elements of vertebrae
3 Amniotic fluid	**17** Ribs
4 Anterior abdominal wall	**18** Skull
5 Biparietal diameter measurement	**19** Spinal canal
6 Cavum septum pellucidum	**20** Spinal cord
7 Cerebellum	**21** Spine
8 Choroid plexus	**22** Stomach
9 Cisterna magna (cerebellomedullary cistern)	**23** Thalamus
	24 Thigh
10 Coronal suture	**25** Umbilical cord
11 Falx cerebri	**26** Umbilical vein
12 Femur	**27** Umbilicus
13 Lambdoid suture	**28** Uterine wall
14 Liver	**29** Vertebral body

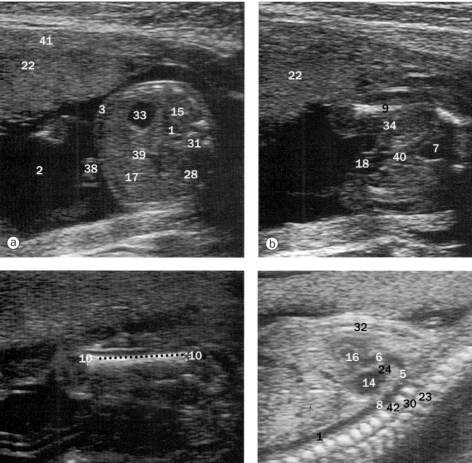

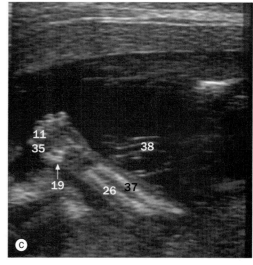

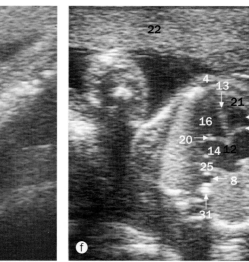

Fetal ultrasound, second trimester:
(a) abdomen, (b) pelvis, (c) forearm,
(d) femur, (e) heart and aorta,
(f) four chamber view of the heart.

1 Abdominal aorta	**22** Placenta
2 Amniotic fluid	**23** Posterior elements of vertebrae
3 Anterior abdominal wall	**24** Pulmonary artery
4 Anterior chest wall	**25** Pulmonary vein
5 Aortic arch	**26** Radius
6 Ascending aorta	**27** Right atrium
7 Bladder	**28** Right kidney
8 Descending aorta	**29** Right ventricle
9 Femur	**30** Spinal canal
10 Femur for femoral length measurement	**31** Spine
11 Finger	**32** Sternum
12 Interatrial septum	**33** Stomach
13 Interventricular septum	**34** Thigh
14 Left atrium	**35** Thumb
15 Left kidney	**36** Tricuspid valve
16 Left ventricle	**37** Ulna
17 Liver	**38** Umbilical cord
18 Male external genitalia	**39** Umbilical vein
19 Metacarpal shaft	**40** Urethra
20 Mitral valve	**41** Uterine wall
21 Moderator band	**42** Vertebral body

7 Lower limb

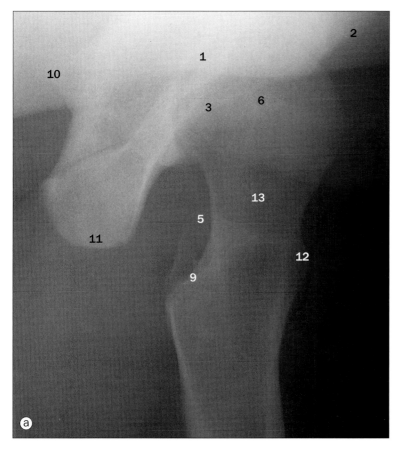

(a) Hip (for neck of femur), lateral projection.

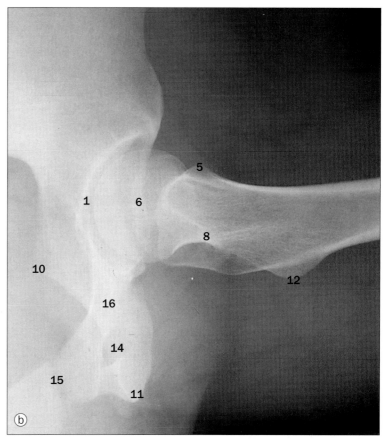

(b) Hip, lateral projection.

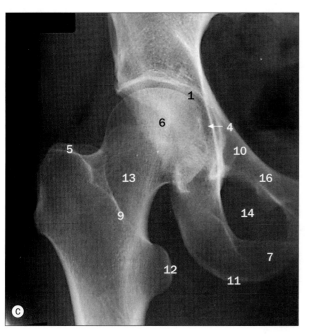

(c) Hip, antero-posterior projection.

1 Acetabulum
2 Anterior inferior iliac spine
3 Epiphysial line
4 Fovea
5 Greater trochanter of femur
6 Head of femur
7 Inferior ramus of pubis
8 Intertrochanteric crest of femur
9 Intertrochanteric line
10 Ischial spine
11 Ischial tuberosity
12 Lesser trochanter of femur
13 Neck of femur
14 Obturator foramen
15 Pubic symphysis
16 Superior ramus of pubis

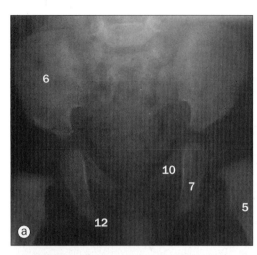

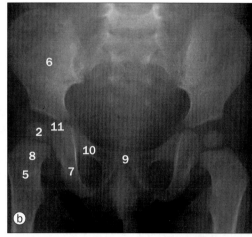

Pelvis, (**a**) of a 2-month-old boy, (**b**) of a 1-year-old boy, (**c**) of an 11-year-old boy, anteroposterior projections.

1	Centre for greater trochanter
2	Centre for head of femur (femoral capital epiphysis)
3	Centre for lesser trochanter
4	Epiphysial line
5	Femur
6	Ilium
7	Ischium
8	Neck of femur
9	Pubic symphysis
10	Pubis
11	Triradiate cartilage
12	Unossified junction between ischium and pubis

INNOMINATE (HIP)	Appears	Fused
Ilium	2–3 miu	7–9 yrs
Ischium	4 miu	7–9 yrs
Pubis	4 miu	7–9 yrs
Acetabulum	11–14 yrs	15–25 yrs
Ant. sup. iliac spine	Puberty	15–25 yrs
Iliac crest/sup. spines	Puberty	15–25 yrs
Ischial tuberosity	Puberty +	15–25 yrs

FEMUR (c)		
Shaft	7 wiu	
Head	4–6 mths	14–18 yrs
Greater trochanter	2–4 yrs	14–18 yrs
Lesser trochanter	10–12 yrs	14–18 yrs
Distal end	9 miu	17–19 yrs

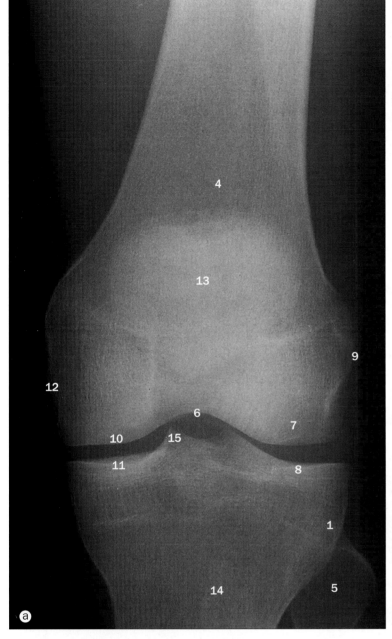

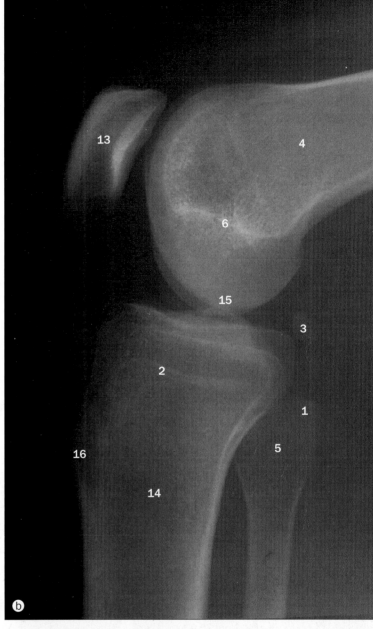

Knee, **(a)** anteroposterior projection, **(b)** lateral projection.
(c) Patella, inferosuperior (skyline) projection.

1	Apex (styloid process) of fibula
2	Epiphysial line
3	Fabella
4	Femur
5	Head of fibula
6	Intercondylar fossa
7	Lateral condyle of femur
8	Lateral condyle of tibia
9	Lateral epicondyle of femur
10	Medial condyle of femur
11	Medial condyle of tibia
12	Medial epicondyle of femur
13	Patella
14	Tibia
15	Tubercles of intercondylar eminence
16	Tuberosity of tibia

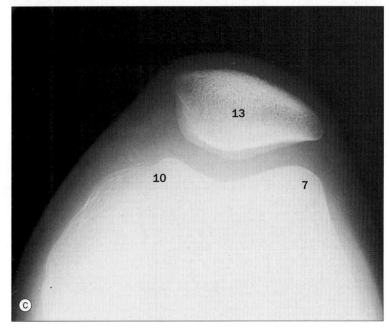

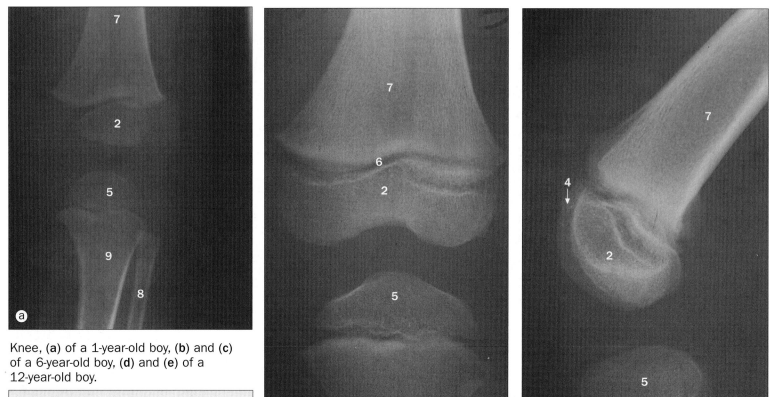

Knee, (**a**) of a 1-year-old boy, (**b**) and (**c**)
of a 6-year-old boy, (**d**) and (**e**) of a
12-year-old boy.

PATELLA (c)	Appears	Fused
1–3 centres	3–5 yrs	Puberty
TIBIA (c)		
Shaft	7 wiu	
Proximal/plateau	9 miu	16–18 yrs
Tuberosity	10–12 yrs	12–14 yrs
Distal end	4 mths–1 yr	15–17 yrs
FIBULA (c)		
Shaft	8 wiu	
Proximal end/head	2–4 yrs	17–19 yrs
Distal end	6 mths–1 yr	15–17 yrs

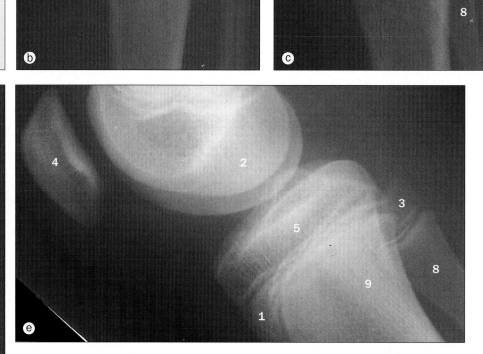

1 Antero-inferior extension of proximal tibial centre for tuberosity of tibia	**5** Centre for proximal tibia
2 Centre for distal femur	**6** Epiphysial line
3 Centre for head of fibula	**7** Femur
4 Centre for patella	**8** Fibula
	9 Tibia

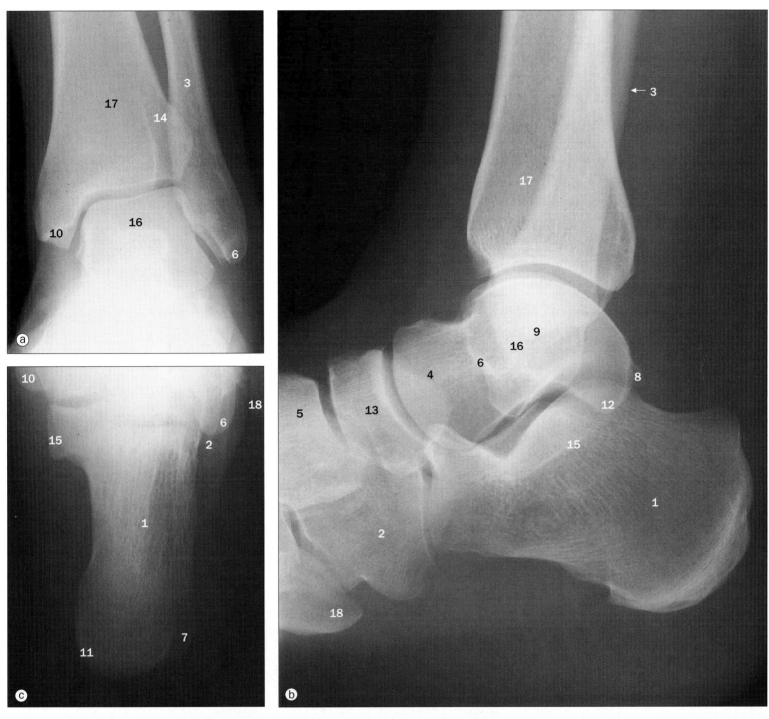

Ankle, (a) anteroposterior projection, (b) lateral projection. (c) Calcaneus, axial projection.

1	Calcaneus	**10**	Medial malleolus of tibia
2	Cuboid	**11**	Medial process of calcaneus
3	Fibula	**12**	Medial tubercle of talus
4	Head of talus	**13**	Navicular
5	Lateral cuneiform	**14**	Region of inferior tibiofibular joint
6	Lateral malleolus of fibula	**15**	Sustentaculum tali of calcaneus
7	Lateral process of calcaneus	**16**	Talus
8	Lateral tubercle of talus	**17**	Tibia
9	Medial malleolus	**18**	Tuberosity of base of fifth metatarsal

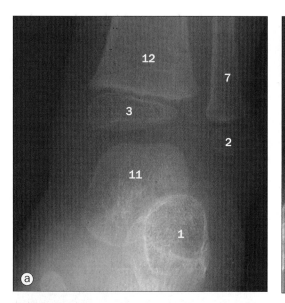

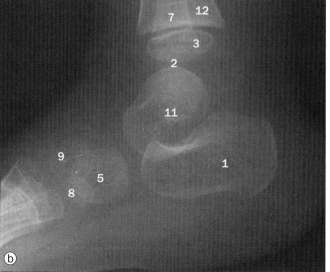

Ankle, (a) and (b) of a
3-year-old boy, (c) and (d)
of a 5-year-old boy, (e) and
(f) of a 13-year-old boy.

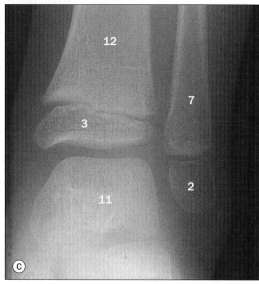

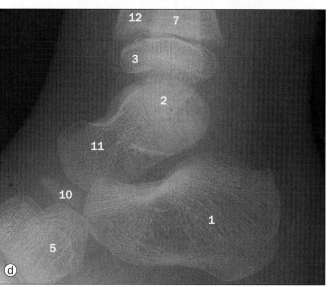

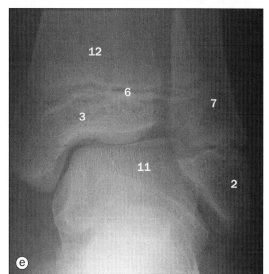

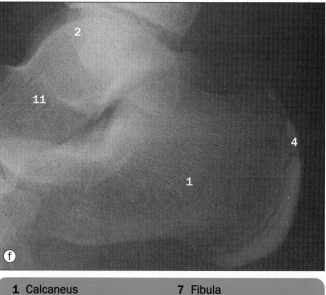

TARSAL BONES (c)	Appears	Fused
Calcaneus	3 miu	14–16 yrs
Talus	6 miu	
Navicular	3 yrs	
Cuneiform lateral	6 mths–1 yr	
Cuneiform intermediate	2–3 yrs	
Cuneiform medial	1–2 yrs	
Cuboid	9 miu	

1	Calcaneus	7	Fibula
2	Centre for distal fibula	8	Intermediate cuneiform
3	Centre for distal tibia	9	Lateral cuneiform
4	Centre for posterior aspect of calcaneus	10	Navicular
5	Cuboid	11	Talus
6	Epiphysial line	12	Tibia

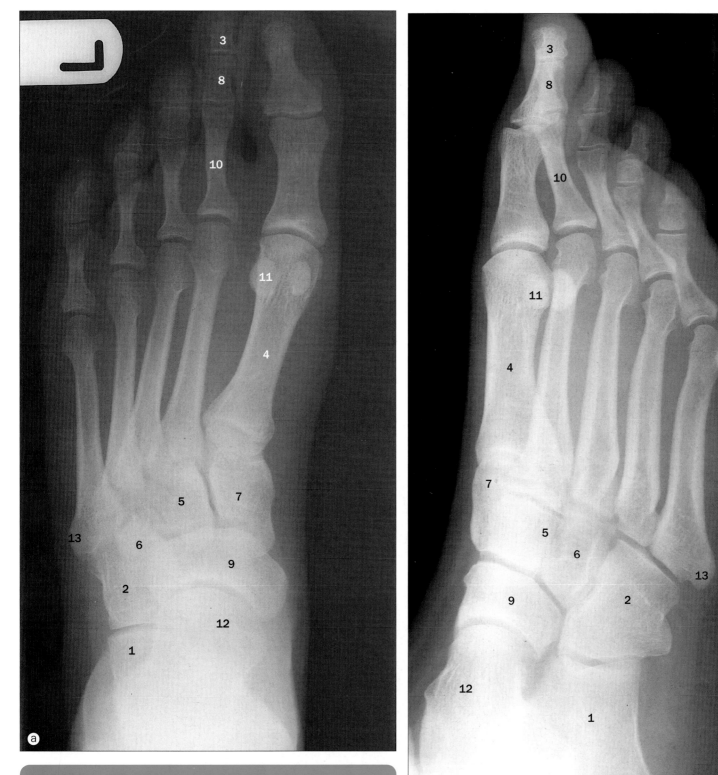

1 Calcaneus
2 Cuboid
3 Distal phalanx of second toe
4 First metatarsal
5 Intermediate cuneiform
6 Lateral cuneiform
7 Medial cuneiform
8 Middle phalanx of second toe
9 Navicular
10 Proximal phalanx of second toe
11 Sesamoid bones in flexor hallucis brevis muscle
12 Talus
13 Tuberosity of base of fifth metatarsal

Foot, (a) dorsoplantar projection, (b) dorsoplantar oblique projection.

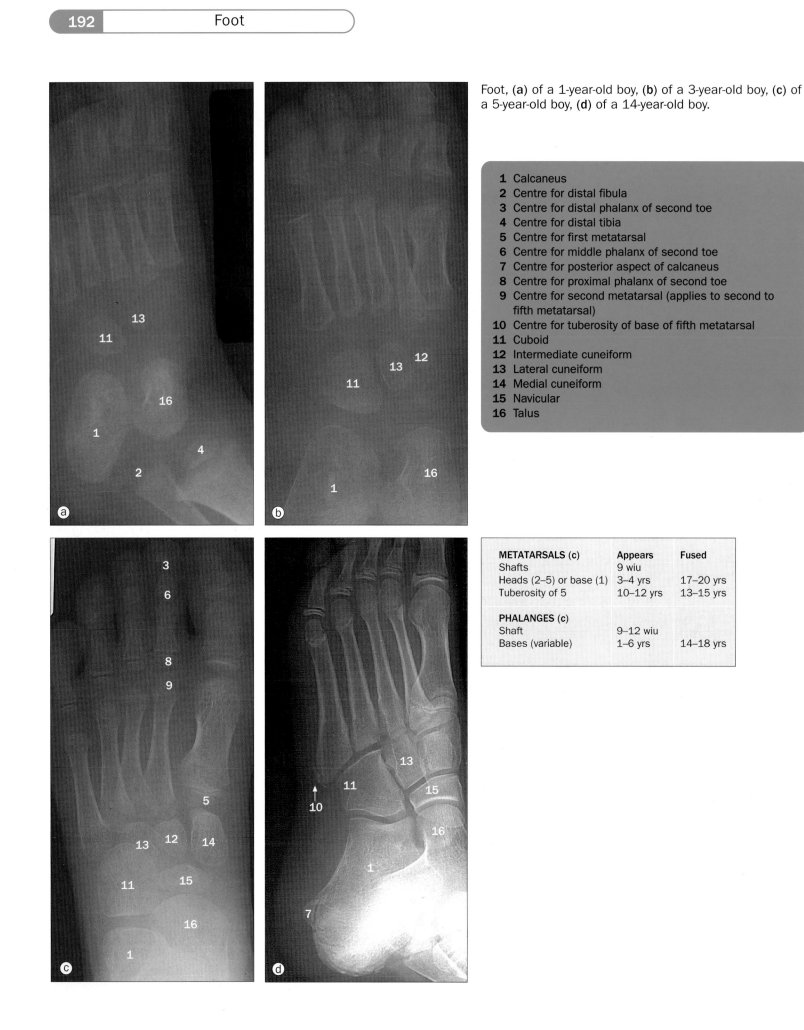

Foot, (a) of a 1-year-old boy, (b) of a 3-year-old boy, (c) of a 5-year-old boy, (d) of a 14-year-old boy.

1 Calcaneus
2 Centre for distal fibula
3 Centre for distal phalanx of second toe
4 Centre for distal tibia
5 Centre for first metatarsal
6 Centre for middle phalanx of second toe
7 Centre for posterior aspect of calcaneus
8 Centre for proximal phalanx of second toe
9 Centre for second metatarsal (applies to second to fifth metatarsal)
10 Centre for tuberosity of base of fifth metatarsal
11 Cuboid
12 Intermediate cuneiform
13 Lateral cuneiform
14 Medial cuneiform
15 Navicular
16 Talus

METATARSALS (c)	Appears	Fused
Shafts	9 wiu	
Heads (2–5) or base (1)	3–4 yrs	17–20 yrs
Tuberosity of 5	10–12 yrs	13–15 yrs

PHALANGES (c)	Appears	Fused
Shaft	9–12 wiu	
Bases (variable)	1–6 yrs	14–18 yrs

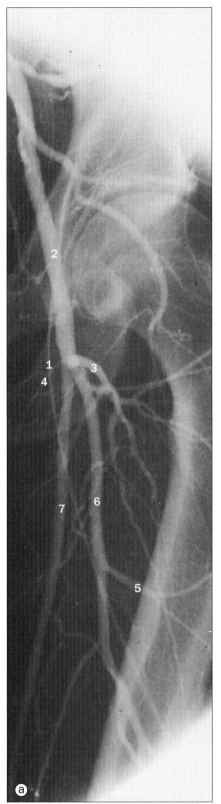

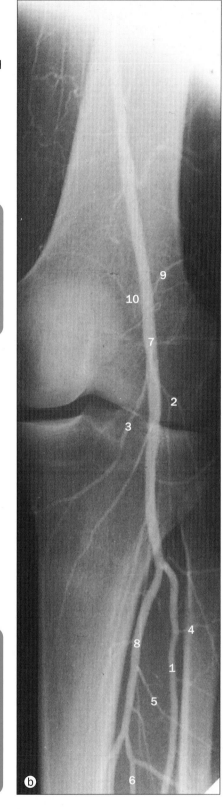

(a) Femoral arteriogram.

The femoropopliteal and tibial arteries are imaged by catheterising the distal abdominal aorta and injecting contrast medium. The column of contrast is then followed as it passes down the legs. If only one leg is to be imaged, an injection into the ipsilateral femoral artery suffices. The external iliac artery continues as the common femoral artery, which originates deep to the inguinal ligament, dividing into the superficial and deep (profunda) femoral arteries. An oblique view is often useful to image the femoral bifurcation and to identify atheroma at the origins of these vessels.

1 Catheter introduced into distal abdominal aorta via left femoral artery
2 Common femoral artery
3 Lateral circumflex femoral artery
4 Medial circumflex femoral artery
5 Perforating artery
6 Profunda femoris artery
7 Superficial femoral artery

(b) Popliteal arteriogram.

The superficial femoral artery becomes the popliteal artery as it passes through the hiatus in the adductor magnus muscle. The popliteal artery terminates at the lower border of the popliteus muscle, dividing into the anterior and posterior tibial arteries.

1 Anterior tibial artery
2 Inferior lateral genicular artery
3 Inferior medial genicular artery
4 Muscular branches of anterior tibial artery
5 Muscular branches of posterior tibial artery
6 Peroneal artery
7 Popliteal artery
8 Posterior tibial artery
9 Superior lateral genicular artery
10 Superior medial genicular artery

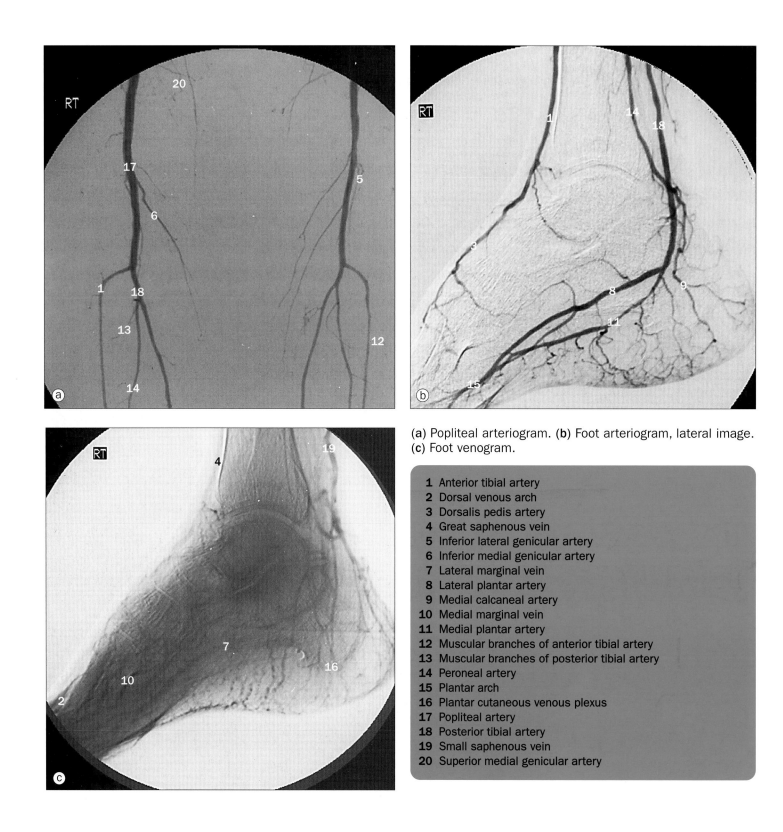

(a) Popliteal arteriogram. (b) Foot arteriogram, lateral image.
(c) Foot venogram.

1 Anterior tibial artery
2 Dorsal venous arch
3 Dorsalis pedis artery
4 Great saphenous vein
5 Inferior lateral genicular artery
6 Inferior medial genicular artery
7 Lateral marginal vein
8 Lateral plantar artery
9 Medial calcaneal artery
10 Medial marginal vein
11 Medial plantar artery
12 Muscular branches of anterior tibial artery
13 Muscular branches of posterior tibial artery
14 Peroneal artery
15 Plantar arch
16 Plantar cutaneous venous plexus
17 Popliteal artery
18 Posterior tibial artery
19 Small saphenous vein
20 Superior medial genicular artery

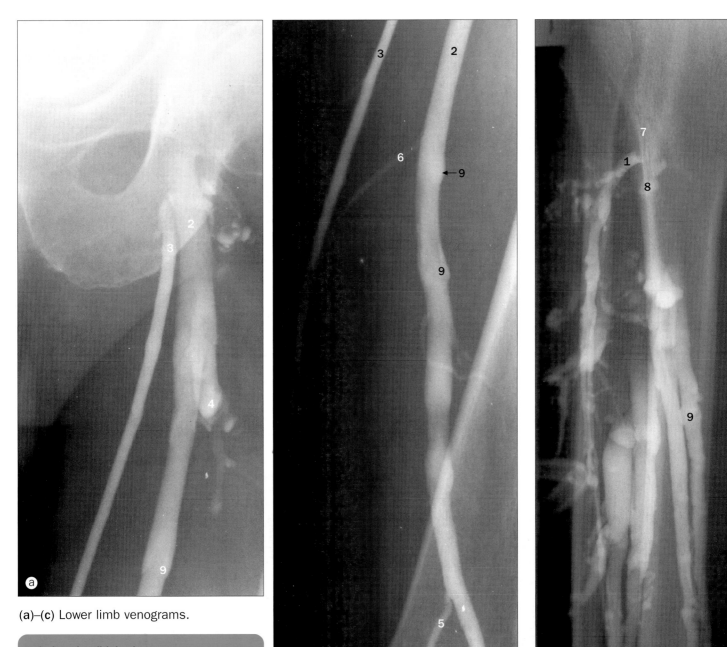

(a)–(c) Lower limb venograms.

1 Anterior tibial vein
2 Femoral vein
3 Great (long) saphenous vein
4 Lateral circumflex vein
5 Muscular tributary of femoral vein
6 Perforating vein
7 Popliteal vein
8 Posterior tibial veins
9 Venous valves

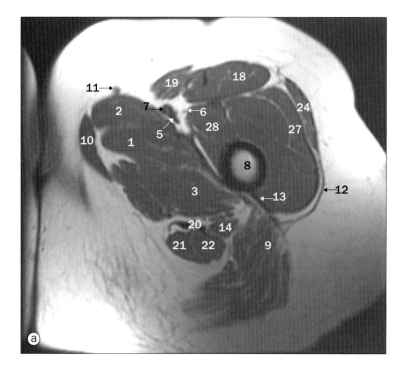

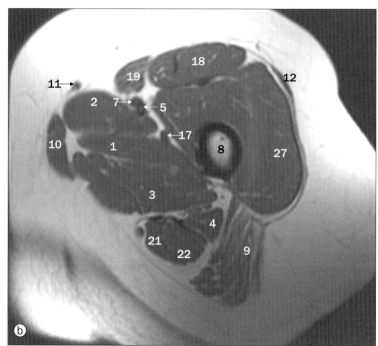

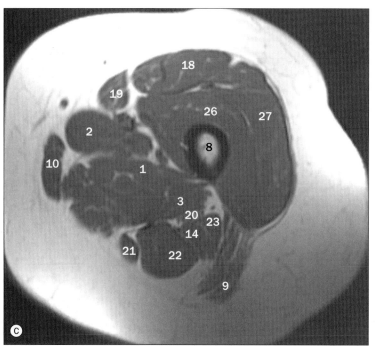

(a)–(f) Thigh, axial MR images

1 Adductor brevis muscle	**9** Gluteus maximus muscle
2 Adductor longus muscle	**10** Gracilis muscle
3 Adductor magnus muscle	**11** Great (long) saphenous vein
4 Biceps femoris muscle	**12** Iliotibial tract
5 Femoral artery	**13** Lateral intermuscular
6 Femoral nerve	septum
7 Femoral vein	**14** Long head of biceps
8 Femur	femoris muscle

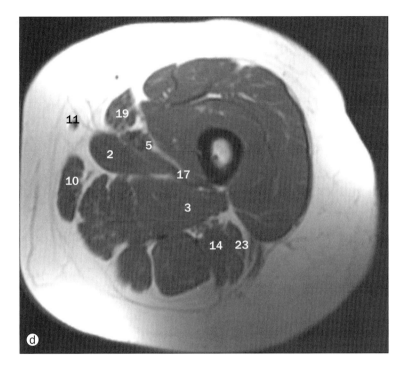

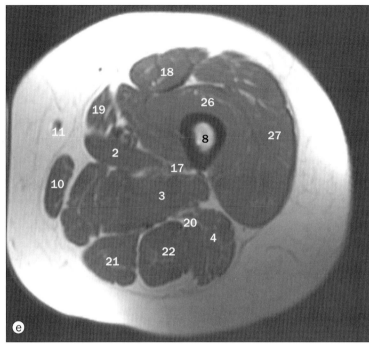

15 Popliteal artery
16 Popliteal vein
17 Profunda femoris artery
18 Rectus femoris muscle
19 Sartorius muscle
20 Sciatic nerve
21 Semimembranosus muscle

22 Semitendinosus muscle
23 Short head of biceps femoris
24 Tensor fasciae latae muscle
25 Tibial nerve
26 Vastus intermedius muscle
27 Vastus lateralis muscle
28 Vastus medialis muscle

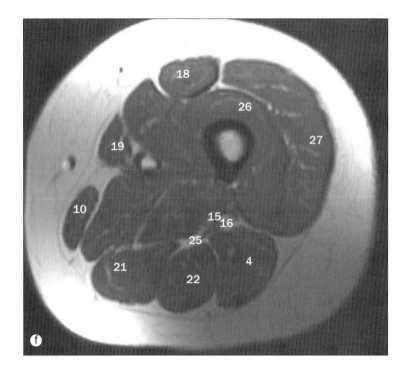

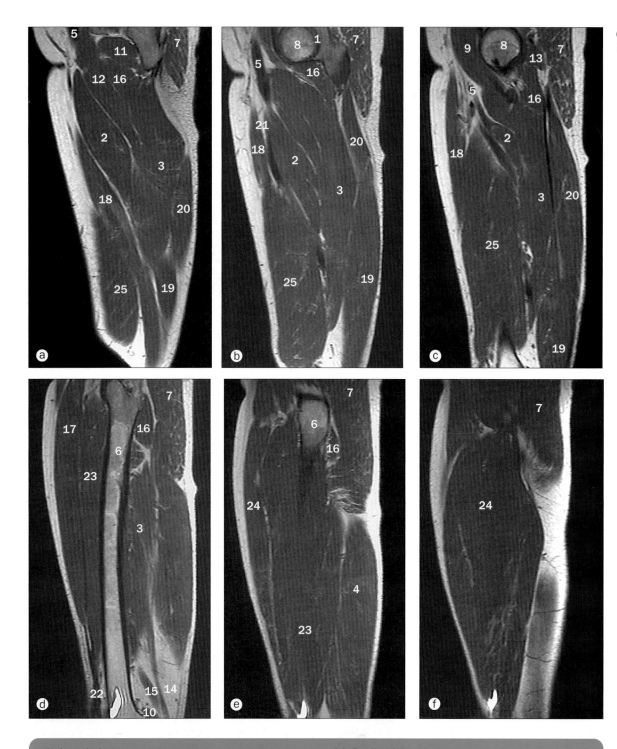

(a)–(f) Thigh, sagittal MR images.

1 Acetabulum	**14** Popliteal artery
2 Adductor longus muscle	**15** Popliteal vein
3 Adductor magnus muscle	**16** Quadratus femoris muscle
4 Biceps femoris muscle	**17** Rectus femoris muscle
5 Femoral artery	**18** Sartorius muscle
6 Femur	**19** Semimembranosus muscle
7 Gluteus maximus muscle	**20** Semitendinosus muscle
8 Head of femur	**21** Subsartorial canal (Hunter's canal)
9 Iliopsoas muscle	**22** Tendon of quadriceps muscle
10 Lateral head of gastrocnemius muscle	**23** Vastus intermedius muscle
11 Obturator externus muscle	**24** Vastus lateralis muscle
12 Pectineus muscle	**25** Vastus medialis muscle
13 Piriformis muscle	

(a)–(f) Thigh, coronal MR images.

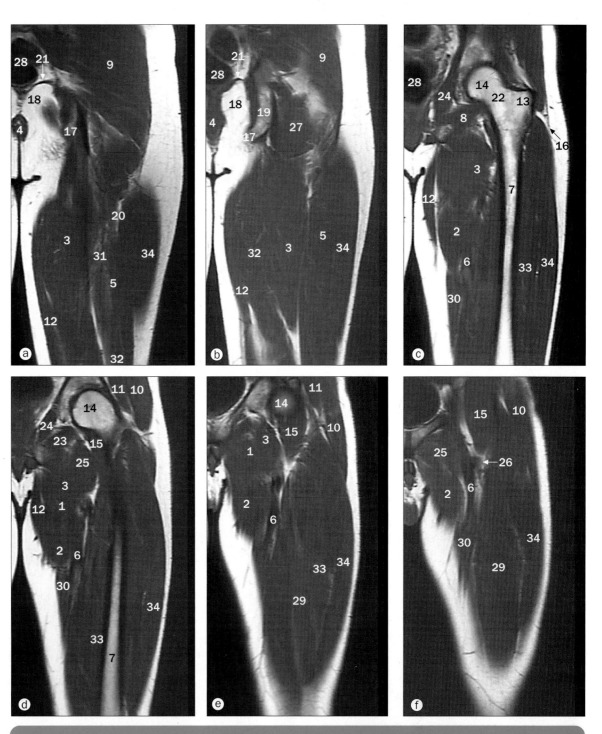

1 Adductor brevis muscle	**18** Ischio-anal fossa
2 Adductor longus muscle	**19** Ischium
3 Adductor magnus muscle	**20** Lateral intermuscular septum
4 Anal canal	**21** Levator ani muscle
5 Biceps femoris muscle	**22** Neck of femur
6 Femoral artery	**23** Obturator externus muscle
7 Femur	**24** Obturator internus muscle
8 Gemellus muscle	**25** Pectineus muscle
9 Gluteus maximus muscle	**26** Profunda femoris artery
10 Gluteus medius muscle	**27** Quadratus femoris muscle
11 Gluteus minimus muscle	**28** Rectum
12 Gracilis muscle	**29** Rectus femoris muscle
13 Greater trochanter of femur	**30** Sartorius muscle
14 Head of femur	**31** Semimembranosus muscle
15 Iliopsoas muscle	**32** Semitendinosus muscle
16 Iliotibial tract	**33** Vastus intermedius muscle
17 Ischial tuberosity	**34** Vastus lateralis muscle

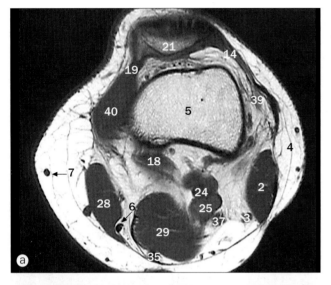

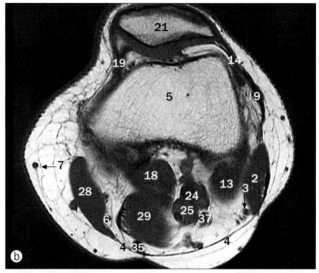

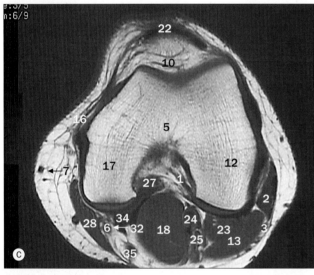

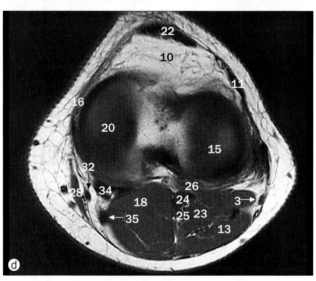

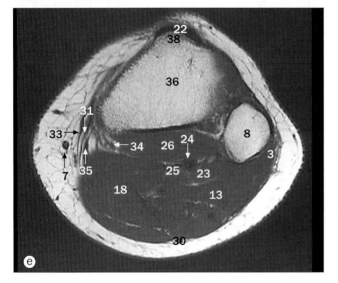

(a)–(e) Knee, axial MR images.

1	Anterior cruciate ligament	**21**	Patella
2	Biceps femoris muscle	**22**	Patellar tendon
3	Common peroneal nerve	**23**	Plantaris muscle
4	Deep fascia of the leg	**24**	Popliteal artery
5	Femur	**25**	Popliteal vein
6	Gracilis muscle	**26**	Popliteus muscle
7	Great saphenous vein	**27**	Posterior cruciate ligament
8	Head of fibula	**28**	Sartorius muscle
9	Iliotibial tract	**29**	Semimembranosus muscle
10	Infrapatellar fat pad	**30**	Short saphenous vein
11	Lateral collateral ligament	**31**	Tendon of gracilis muscle
12	Lateral condyle of femur	**32**	Tendon of gracilis muscle
13	Lateral head of gastrocnemius muscle	**33**	Tendon of sartorius muscle
14	Lateral patellar retinaculum	**34**	Tendon of semimembranosus muscle
15	Lateral tibial plateau	**35**	Tendon of semitendinosus muscle
16	Medial collateral ligament		
17	Medial condyle of femur	**36**	Tibia
18	Medial head of gastrocnemius muscle	**37**	Tibial nerve
		38	Tibial tubercle
19	Medial patellar retinaculum	**39**	Vastus lateralis muscle
20	Medial tibial plateau	**40**	Vastus medialis muscle

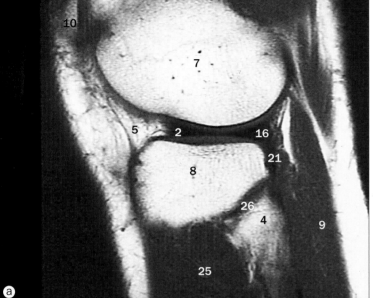

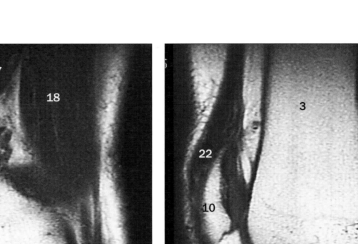

(a)–(c) Knee, sagittal MR images.

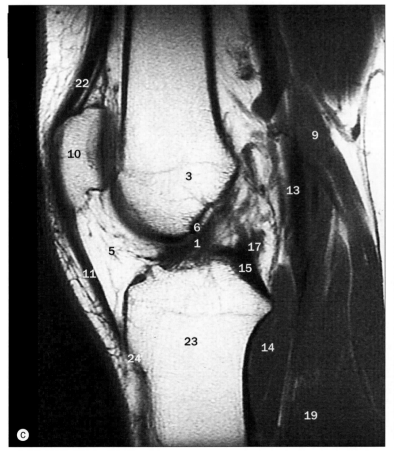

1 Anterior cruciate ligament
2 Anterior horn of lateral meniscus
3 Femur
4 Head of fibula
5 Infrapatellar fat pad
6 Intercondylar notch
7 Lateral condyle of femur
8 Lateral condyle of tibia
9 Lateral head of gastrocnemius muscle
10 Patella
11 Patellar tendon
12 Plantaris muscle
13 Popliteal artery and vein
14 Popliteus muscle
15 Posterior cruciate ligament
16 Posterior horn of lateral meniscus
17 Posterior meniscofemoral ligament
18 Short head of biceps femoris muscle
19 Soleus muscle
20 Superior lateral genicular artery
21 Tendon of popliteus muscle
22 Tendon of quadriceps muscle
23 Tibia
24 Tibial tubercle
25 Tibialis anterior muscle
26 Tibiofibular joint
27 Vastus lateralis muscle

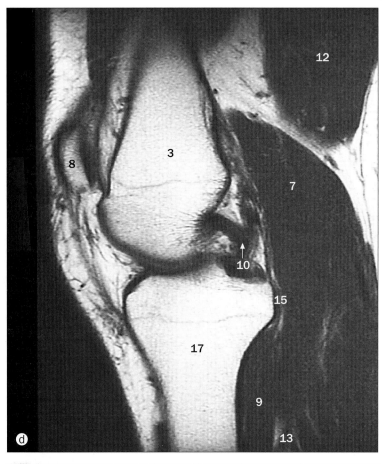

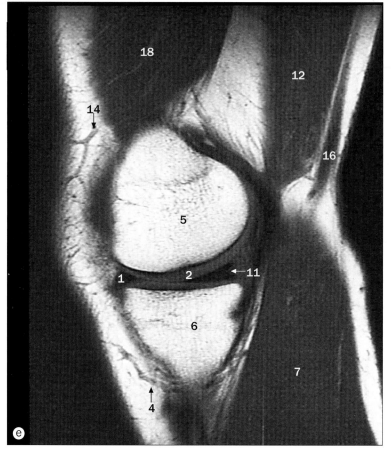

(d)–(f) Knee, sagittal MR images.

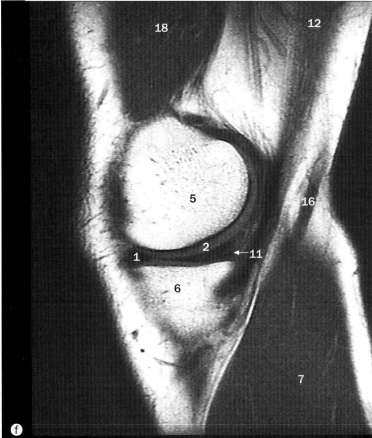

1 Anterior horn of medial meniscus
2 Articular cartilage
3 Femur
4 Inferior medial genicular artery
5 Medial condyle of femur
6 Medial condyle of tibia
7 Medial head of gastrocnemius muscle
8 Patella
9 Popliteus muscle
10 Posterior cruciate ligament
11 Posterior horn of medial meniscus
12 Semimembranosus muscle
13 Soleus muscle
14 Superior medial genicular artery
15 Tendon of popliteus muscle
16 Tendon of semitendinosus muscle
17 Tibia
18 Vastus medialis muscle

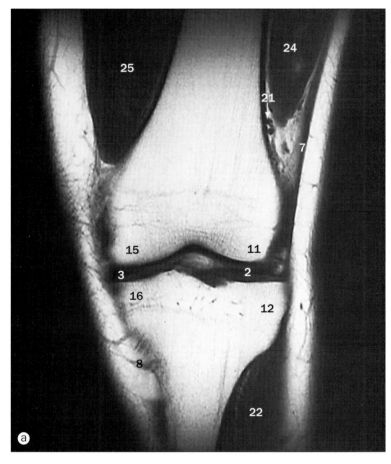

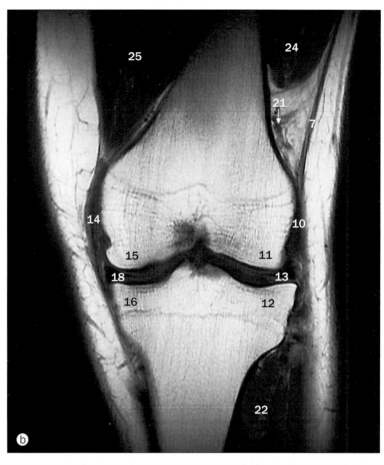

(a)–(f) Knee, coronal MR images.

1 Anterior cruciate ligament
2 Anterior horn of lateral meniscus
3 Anterior horn of medial meniscus
4 Biceps femoris muscle
5 Great (long) saphenous vein
6 Head of fibula
7 Iliotibial tract
8 Inferior medial genicular artery
9 Intercondylar notch
10 Lateral collateral ligament
11 Lateral condyle of femur
12 Lateral condyle of tibia
13 Lateral meniscus
14 Medial collateral ligament
15 Medial condyle of femur
16 Medial condyle of tibia
17 Medial head of gastrocnemius muscle
18 Medial meniscus
19 Posterior cruciate ligament
20 Sartorius muscle
21 Superior lateral genicular artery
22 Tibialis anterior muscle
23 Tibiofibular joint
24 Vastus lateralis muscle
25 Vastus medialis muscle

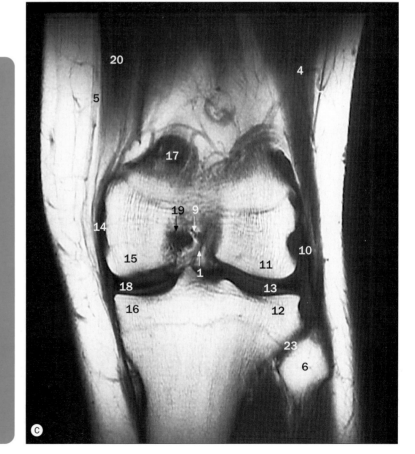

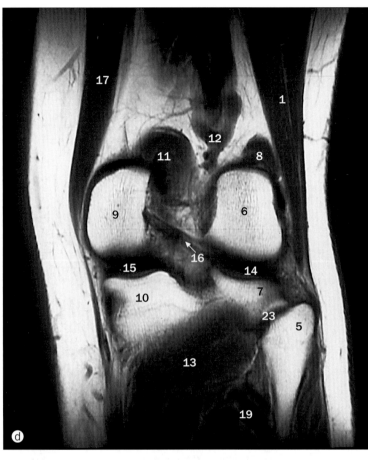

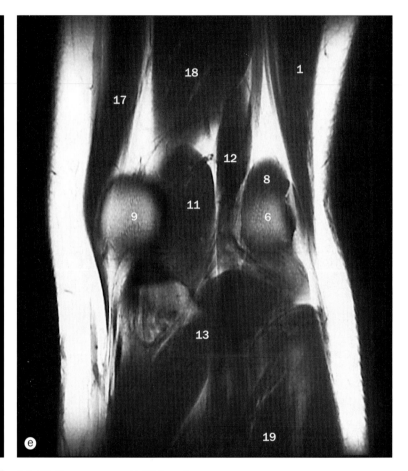

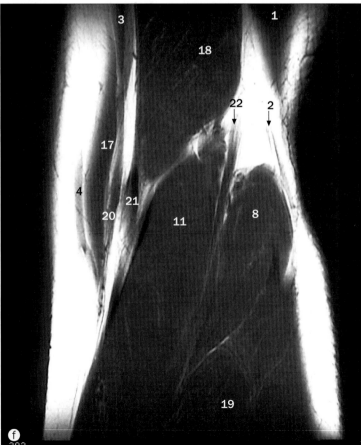

(d)–(f) Knee, coronal MR images.

1 Biceps femoris muscle
2 Common peroneal nerve
3 Gracilis muscle
4 Great (long) saphenous vein
5 Head of fibula
6 Lateral condyle of femur
7 Lateral condyle of tibia
8 Lateral head of gastrocnemius muscle
9 Medial condyle of femur
10 Medial condyle of tibia
11 Medial head of gastrocnemius muscle
12 Popliteal artery and vein
13 Popliteus muscle
14 Posterior horn of lateral meniscus
15 Posterior horn of medial meniscus
16 Posterior meniscofemoral ligament
17 Sartorius muscle
18 Semimembranosus muscle
19 Soleus muscle
20 Tendon of gracilis muscle
21 Tendon of semitendinosus muscle
22 Tibial nerve
23 Tibiofibular joint

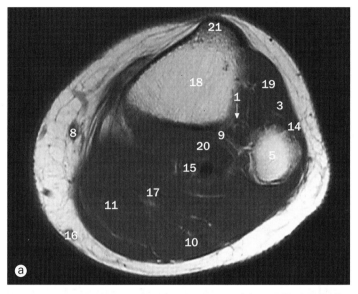

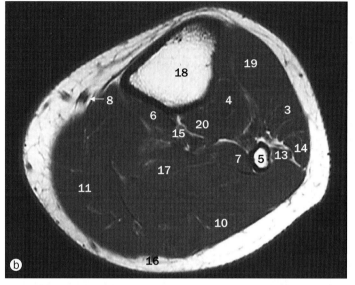

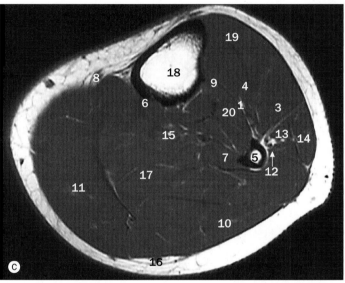

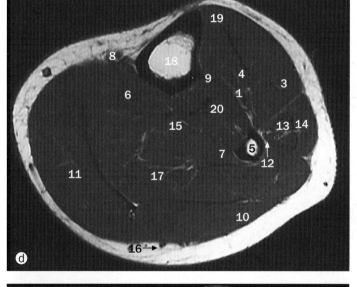

(a)–(e) Calf, axial MR images.

1 Anterior tibial artery
2 Aponeurosis of gastrocnemius muscle
3 Extensor digitorum longus muscle
4 Extensor hallucis longus muscle
5 Fibula
6 Flexor digitorum longus muscle
7 Flexor hallucis longus muscle
8 Great (long) saphenous vein
9 Interosseous membrane
10 Lateral head of gastrocnemius muscle
11 Medial head of gastrocnemius muscle
12 Peroneal artery
13 Peroneus brevis muscle
14 Peroneus longus muscle
15 Posterior tibial artery
16 Small saphenous vein
17 Soleus muscle
18 Tibia
19 Tibialis anterior muscle
20 Tibialis posterior muscle
21 Tuberosity of tibia

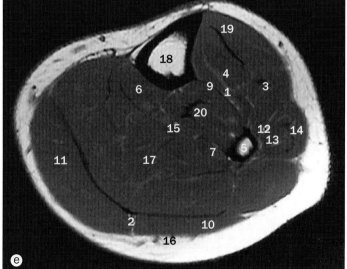

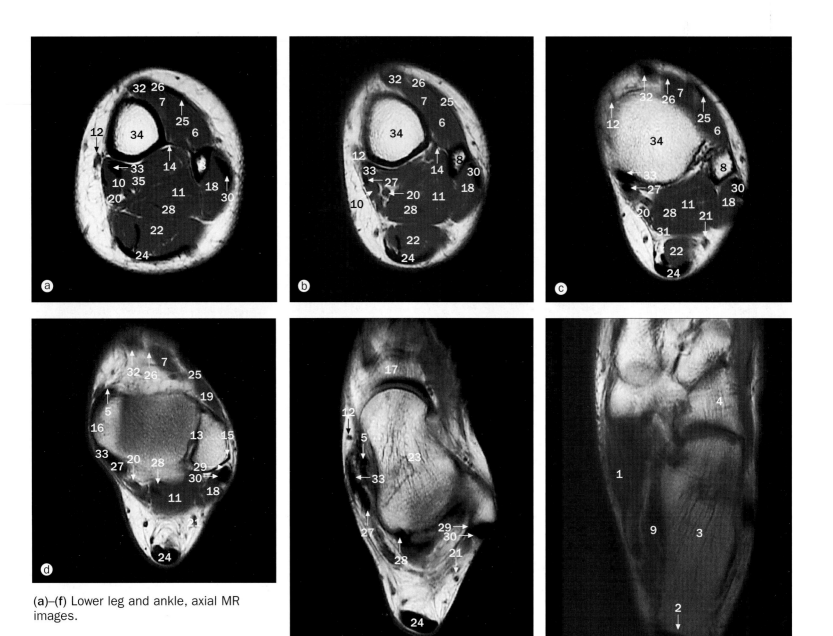

(a)–(f) Lower leg and ankle, axial MR images.

1 Abductor hallucis muscle	**19** Peroneus tertius muscle
2 Calcaneal tuberosity	**20** Posterior tibial artery and vein
3 Calcaneus	**21** Small saphenous vein
4 Cuboid	**22** Soleus muscle
5 Deltoid ligament	**23** Talus
6 Extensor digitorum muscle	**24** Tendo calcaneus (Achilles' tendon)
7 Extensor hallucis longus muscle	**25** Tendon of extensor digitorum muscle
8 Fibula	**26** Tendon of extensor hallucis longus muscle
9 Flexor accessorius muscle	**27** Tendon of flexor digitorum longus muscle
10 Flexor digitorum longus muscle	**28** Tendon of flexor hallucis longus muscle
11 Flexor hallucis longus muscle	**29** Tendon of peroneus brevis muscle
12 Great (long) saphenous vein	**30** Tendon of peroneus longus muscle
13 Inferior tibiofibular joint	**31** Tendon of plantaris muscle
14 Interosseous membrane	**32** Tendon of tibialis anterior muscle
15 Lateral malleolus	**33** Tendon of tibialis posterior muscle
16 Medial malleolus	**34** Tibia
17 Navicular	**35** Tibialis posterior muscle
18 Peroneus brevis muscle	

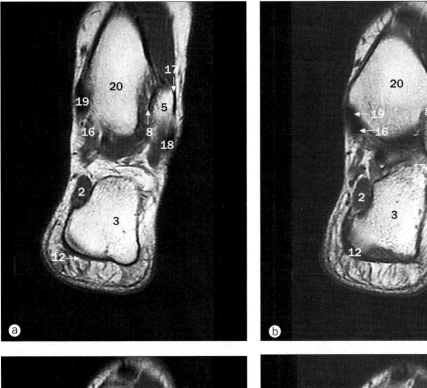

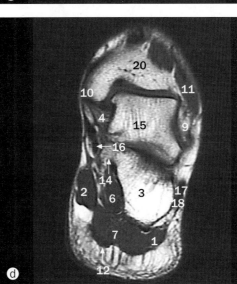

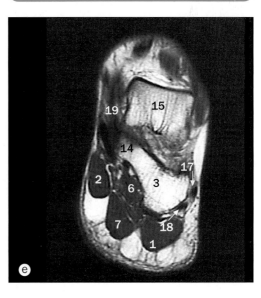

(a)–(e) Foot, axial MR images..

1 Abductor digiti minimi muscle
2 Abductor hallucis muscle
3 Calcaneus
4 Deltoid ligament
5 Fibula
6 Flexor accessorius muscle
7 Flexor digitorum brevis muscle
8 Inferior tibiofibular joint
9 Lateral malleolus
10 Medial malleolus
11 Peroneus tertius muscle
12 Plantar aponeurosis
13 Posterior tibial artery
14 Sustentaculum tali
15 Talus
16 Tendon of flexor digitorum longus muscle
17 Tendon of peroneus brevis muscle
18 Tendon of peroneus longus muscle
19 Tendon of tibialis posterior muscle
20 Tibia

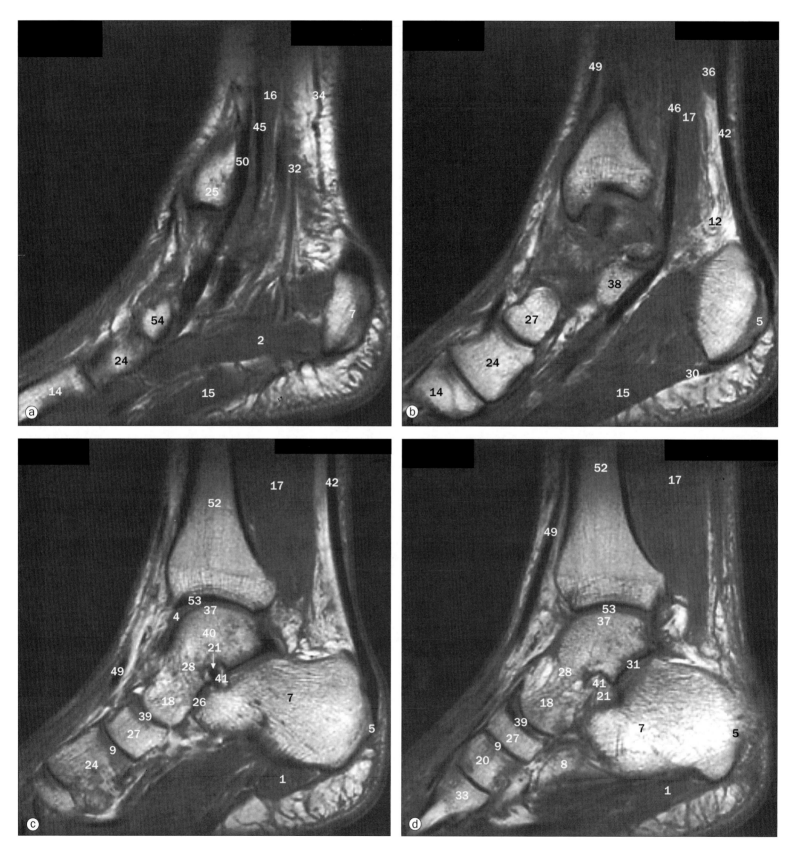

(a)–(f) Ankle, sagittal MR images.

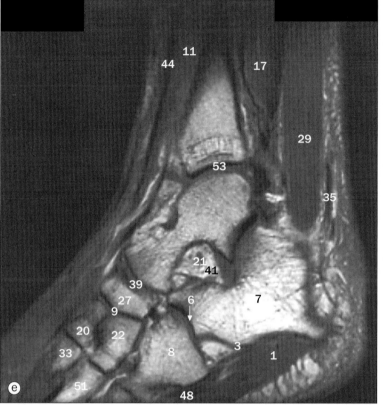

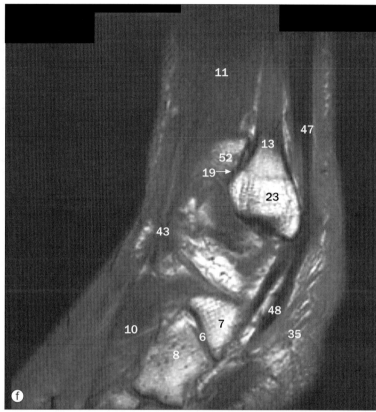

1 Abductor digiti minimi muscle	**19** Inferior tibiofibular joint	**37** Superior surface of talus
2 Abductor hallucis muscle	**20** Intermediate cuneiform	**38** Sustentaculum tali
3 Anterior tubercle of calcaneus	**21** Interosseous talocalcaneal ligament	**39** Talonavicular joint
4 Articular cartilage	**22** Lateral cuneiform	**40** Talus
5 Calcaneal tuberosity	**23** Lateral malleolus	**41** Tarsal sinus
6 Calcaneocuboid joint	**24** Medial cuneiform	**42** Tendo calcaneus (Achilles' tendon)
7 Calcaneus	**25** Medial malleolus	**43** Tendon of extensor digitorum muscle
8 Cuboid	**26** Medial subtalar joint	**44** Tendon of extensor hallucis longus muscle
9 Cuneonavicular joint	**27** Navicular	**45** Tendon of flexor digitorum longus muscle
10 Extensor digitorum brevis muscle	**28** Neck of talus	**46** Tendon of flexor hallucis longus muscle
11 Extensor digitorum muscle	**29** Peroneus brevis muscle	**47** Tendon of peroneus brevis muscle
12 Fat pad	**30** Plantar aponeurosis	**48** Tendon of peroneus longus muscle
13 Fibula	**31** Posterior subtalar joint	**49** Tendon of tibialis anterior muscle
14 First metatarsal	**32** Posterior tibial artery and vein	**50** Tendon of tibialis posterior muscle
15 Flexor digitorum brevis muscle	**33** Second metatarsal	**51** Third metatarsal
16 Flexor digitorum longus muscle	**34** Short saphenous vein	**52** Tibia
17 Flexor hallucis longus muscle	**35** Small saphenous vein	**53** Tibiotalar part of ankle joint
18 Head of talus	**36** Soleus muscle	**54** Tuberosity of navicular

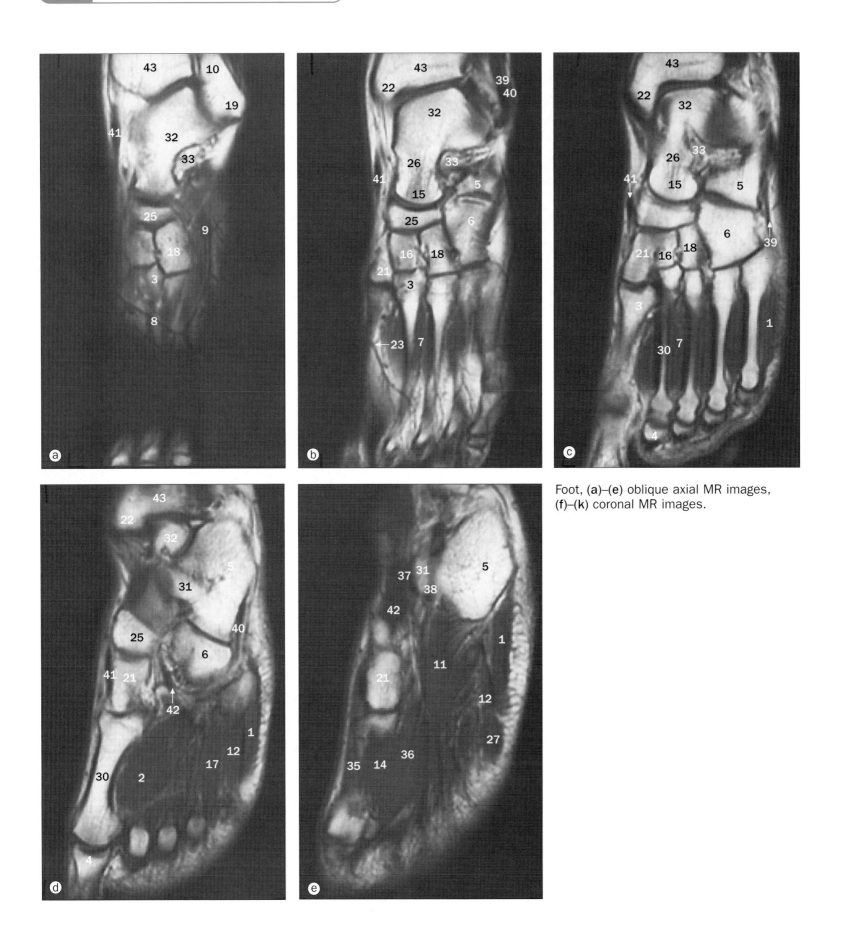

Foot, (a)–(e) oblique axial MR images, (f)–(k) coronal MR images.

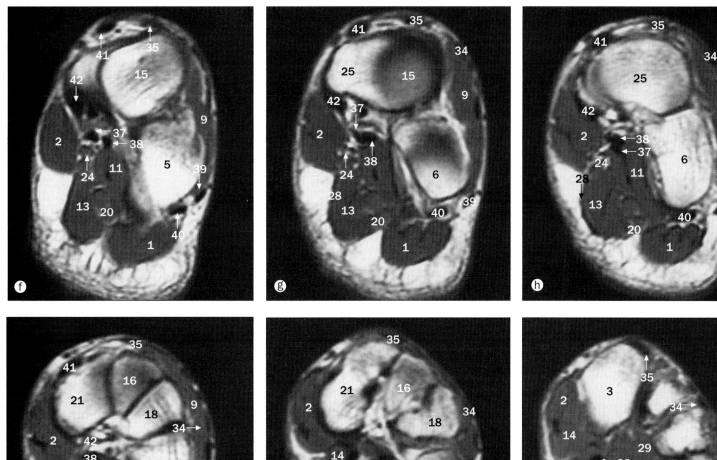

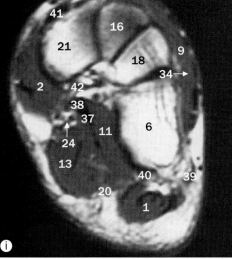

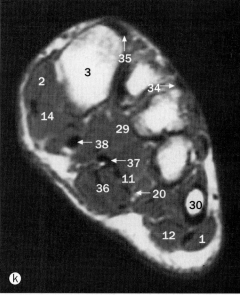

1 Abductor digiti minimi muscle	**23** Medial marginal vein
2 Adductor hallucis muscle	**24** Medial plantar nerve and artery
3 Base of metatarsal	**25** Navicular
4 Base of proximal phalanx	**26** Neck of talus
5 Calcaneus	**27** Opponens digiti minimi muscle
6 Cuboid	**28** Plantar aponeurosis
7 Dorsal interossei muscle	**29** Plantar interossei muscle
8 Dorsal venous arch	**30** Shaft of metatarsal
9 Extensor digitorum brevis muscle	**31** Sustentaculum tali
10 Fibula	**32** Talus
11 Flexor accessorius muscle	**33** Tarsal sinus
12 Flexor digiti minimi muscle	**34** Tendon of extensor digitorum longus muscle
13 Flexor digitorum brevis muscle	**35** Tendon of extensor hallucis longus muscle
14 Flexor hallucis brevis muscle	**36** Tendon of flexor digitorum brevis muscle
15 Head of talus	**37** Tendon of flexor digitorum longus muscle
16 Intermediate cuneiform	**38** Tendon of flexor hallucis longus muscle
17 Interossei muscles	**39** Tendon of peroneus brevis muscle
18 Lateral cuneiform	**40** Tendon of peroneus longus muscle
19 Lateral malleolus	**41** Tendon of tibialis anterior muscle
20 Lateral plantar nerve	**42** Tendon of tibialis posterior muscle
21 Medial cuneiform	**43** Tibia
22 Medial malleolus	

Index